MW01078241

Works of Illness
Narrative, Picturing and the
Social Response to Serious Disease

Alan Radley

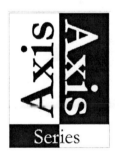

Series

InkerMen Press
2009

Works of Illness
Narrative, Picturing and the Social Response to Serious Disease
by
Alan Radley

Copyright © Alan Radley 2009

This edition first published in 2009
Copyright © InkerMen Press 2009

Front Cover: Photograph © Ian Robertson, *"Stefan Wahrlich"*, 1998.
Courtesy R. and J. Watson Trust and the Cancer Society of New Zealand.
www.ianrobertson.co.nz

Back Cover: Photograph © The Jo Spence Memorial Archive,
Jo Spence "Looking Death in the Eye", The Final Project, 1991,
Courtesy Terry Dennett, London.

InkerMen Press
Ashby-de-la-Zouch
info@inkermenpress.co.uk
www.inkermenpress.co.uk

978-0-9562749-0-8

The Axis Series Volume 8
Series Editor: Daniel Watt

British Library Cataloguing in Publication Data

Radley, Alan, 1946-
    Works of illness : narrative, picturing and the social
    response to serious disease. – (The axis series ; v. 8)
    1. Social medicine. 2. Sick in literature. 3. Sick in art.
    I. Title II. Series
    306.4'61-dc22

ISBN-13: 9780956274908

Works of Illness
Narrative, Picturing and the
Social Response to Serious Disease

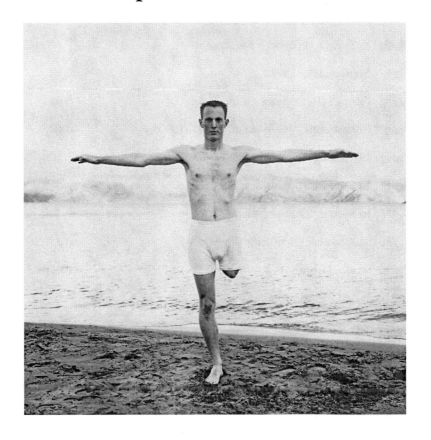

Alan Radley

List of Figures

Contents

Author's Note

This book is the outcome of work that I have published in several articles and chapters over the past ten years. I draw upon, and in part reproduce in this text sections from the following articles: in Chapter 5 and 6, Radley, A., The aesthetics of illness: narrative, horror and the sublime, *Sociology of Health & Illness*, 1999, 21 (6), 778-796; Radley, A. and Taylor, D., Images of recovery: a photo-elicitation study on the hospital ward, *Qualitative Health Research*, 2003, 13 (1), 77-99. In Chapters 2 and 4, Radley, A. and Bell, S.E., Artworks, collective experience and claims for social justice: the case of women living with breast cancer. *Sociology of Health & Illness*, 2007, 29 (3) 366-390. I am indebted to Susan Bell for allowing me to use this jointly written text. Chapters 4 and 5 include excerpts from Radley, A. Portrayals of suffering: on looking away, looking at, and the comprehension of illness experience, *Body & Society*, 2002, 8 (3), 1-23.

For Margaret, Lisa, Kate and Dan, and Isaac – my family.

Acknowledgements

In the years leading up to writing this book I have benefited from many talks with friends and colleagues about illness and its representation. Arthur Frank has been especially supportive and generous, both as someone who has written about his own illness and as a focus for work on illness narratives. Susan Bell provided me with the opportunity to work with the artist's books of Martha Hall held at Bowdoin College, and more important, the chance for us to work together on questions of visual representation of illness experience. I am especially grateful to Susan for allowing me to quote at length from our joint paper on 'Artworks' in Chapter 2 of this book. Terry Dennett has been unstinting in his generosity with photographs taken by both him and Jo Spence, and in providing valuable information about their work together. The thinking behind the present book owes much to conversations with various colleagues over the years – including members of the "Narrative Group" in Boston – Elliot Mishler, Cathy Riessman, Arlene Katz, Brinton Lykes, and Susan Bell. On the subject of illness narratives, Rita Charon has been an inspiration in her work, as has David Morris, who kindly invited me to meetings in San Diego and in Bellagio so that my ideas got a 'run-out' with experts from other fields. An invitation from Kerry Chamberlain and John Spicer to visit Massey University, New Zealand in 1998 gave me the time and space to sketch out some early ideas that find their fruition in these pages – to both of them I remain deeply grateful. While in New Zealand I attended an exhibition of portraits and stories about cancer patients, organised by Halina Ogonowska-Coates with photographs by Ian Robertson, both of whom I thank for allowing me to reproduce the photograph of Stefan Wahrlich. I thank Stefan Wahrlich and Elissa Aleshire for allowing their portraits to appear in this book.

I am also grateful to those organizations who have allowed me to reproduce images for which they hold copyright, including The Breast Cancer Fund of America; The Jo Spence Memorial Archive, London; The Robert Pope Foundation, Nova Scotia, Canada; Alan Hall and the George J. Mitchell Department of Special Collections & Archives, Bowdoin College Library, Brunswick, Maine; Ronald Feldman Fine Arts, New York; and the Minneapolis Institute of Arts, The Ethel Morrison Van Derlip Fund.

Art is a revolt against fate.

André Malraux, *Voices of Silence*

Introduction

The origins of this book lie in a research study that I carried out in the 1980s with men who had received bypass surgery to relieve chest pain associated with coronary artery disease. In particular, two men told us how they dealt with their illness in the months following surgery, one by digging his garden and the other by chopping wood in his shed. Both men relished the fact that they did this in spite of their wives' disapproval, given that they had been told to take things carefully by the doctors. More important, though, was that the men felt that only by acting in this way could they demonstrate to their wives (and, I assumed to other people, including the researchers) that they were on the road to recovery. This dramatisation of everyday activity was a performance that showed they were well again, adding to any verbal claims that they might make about their recovered state of health. Not only in the doing of these things, but in the telling, the men showed that the recovery of health was something that had to be given some shape, done with some style if it was to be accepted by other people. It was not just that they could do these everyday jobs once more. The men did so (they said) almost theatrically, in the sight of their wives who, in their turn, told us that they did not approve, at least initially. Of course, gardens were successfully dug and wood got chopped, but these matters were by themselves not a key to understanding what was going on here. The important things were the nature of the performance, the role of the wives as protagonists, and the witnessing of the whole event at second hand through the men's storytelling at interview. These things gave their actions a wider claim to a style of recovery – an act, almost, of recovery through imagination.

While all the patients we spoke to did not give similar accounts, I concluded that what these two men did could be seen as being prototypical of how anybody with a serious illness might express their state of health. What struck me was that these performances *worked* for the men, in that they said that, through these actions, they re-claimed something important about their world; they *worked*, albeit perversely at times, for the wives who came to see a future relationship with their husbands beyond the demands of illness; and they *worked* for us, the researchers, through the stories that conveyed something of the performances concerned. And all this from acts of digging and chopping that, though mundane in their effects, were also embellishments, copies of 'the real thing'. Whatever worked for the men (they said they felt better), eventually for the wives, and ultimately for us, as researchers, needed explaining. What sort of work was involved here? What did it produce? If the men's labours made something lasting beyond turned soil or chopped wood, what was that likely to be? This book takes up these questions in a context where the product of people's efforts attains a tangible, social form, issuing in artefacts made to represent what it means to live with illness that is debilitating and sometimes life-threatening.

A good performance, done with style, is an aesthetic act. By this I mean that it has qualities – however fleeting – that counter the uncertainty and horror that often accompanies serious disease. Aesthetic features do not figure highly in medical sociology or health psychology, though they do, perhaps unexpectedly, in medicine itself. This might be because medicine is a practice as well as a discipline, and the idea of good practice inevitably raises issues of ethics. In this book I discuss representations of life with illness – especially those made in published accounts and pictures – in terms of both aesthetics and ethics, as well as in terms of ideologies and social action. In doing this I steer a course between the positions of the philosophy of art, ethics and medical sociology, without ever adhering to one alone. For that reason, this book does not sit easily within a medical sociology that has no place for aesthetics, in an appreciation of art that is unconcerned with ethics, or in a discussion of bioethics that has little concern for the material world. While other books might be written specifically about 'the art of illness representations', or 'the ethics of illness representations' or 'the social context of illness representations', none, in my view, can satisfactorily address questions of how pictures and stories made by ill people do their work. In consequence, this book trades on and between these positions, borrows here and lends there, as I believe it must if it is to do *its work*.

I have chosen to discuss accounts written and pictures made by ill people who do these things with the skill of the artist. (Several of them were artists.) The reason for this is that I want to explore, in as clear a way as possible, how these artefacts make meaning, are used in organising social action and serve as a medium for survival. I could discern this in the labours of the men digging gardens and chopping wood, but could not describe its genesis or consequences. This was because their actions were too fleeting, having insufficient form that I could hold on to. I needed something longer-lasting, something one might say that 'stands up on its own'. Addressing artefacts like published stories and pictures allows sufficient time and space to describe the role of protagonists and witnesses, and to discuss the role of researchers in how such representations operate.

For a similar reason – to do with tangibility and with ascetic distance – I did not want to use as my focus what is generally known as 'art therapy', where the works would be less easy to place in terms of social context. Readers who are practitioners and researchers involved in art therapy will, I hope, bear with me on this limitation to my argument.

One outstanding question is, can one evaluate the role of stories (narratives) and pictures (visual material) in the same way? Are they indeed separable, or do they trade on one another in ways that require some unifying conceptual framework? I have done my best in this book to bring to bear upon narrative and visual material some concepts that I believe illuminate both. In order to do this I have drawn heavily – and with gratitude – upon the work of scholars in the fields of narrative, of visual studies and philosophy. Rather than try to fashion some conceptual scheme that covers all representation, I have reserved my arguments for questions to do with serious illness, its understanding and the social response it provokes. For that reason this book is best thought of as an attempt to widen the arguments about what it means to be ill in the modern world, where that condition has become part of a wider debate about how to live well with disease that is only partly overcome or that leaves social as well as bodily scars.

What I half knew back then, when I talked to the men with heart disease, but know more clearly now is that when people fall ill they resort to whatever they have in their lives – their skills, resources, their relationships – to make sense of the future they have or, in some cases, have left. Only for a relatively few people, perhaps, will this involve writing and publishing accounts, painting pictures or making photographs. And yet the aims of recovering the ability to wonder, to help others see clearly – perhaps for the first time – how things might be, are always at the centre of efforts to shape life in the face of illness. Describing and explaining these efforts is what this book attempts to do.

Chapter 1

Ethics, Aesthetics, and the Representation of Illness Experience

With the benefits of treatment for serious disease there appears alongside new technologies the question of how to live with the uncertainties that a chronic illness can bring. The deeper that medicine reaches inside the body, either to cure or to investigate, it raises questions about the effects of diagnosis, prognosis and treatment in the lives of patients and those around them. This involves making sense of the kind of person one has become or could be in the shadow of a condition that might remain or worsen. We might say that the therapeutic benefits of modern medicine create in each survivor a nodal point in which everyday experience is provoked. Deciding what is healthy (in the sense of a return to good health) might not be the sole or appropriate objective any more. Instead, how to achieve a sense of well-being, and with that a sense of personal and collective worth, becomes a primary aim.

Where people move from being mere survivors to being witnesses of suffering and treatment, then it appears that the everyday reaches back to embrace others, both outside of and inside medicine. This defines the territory of an 'ethics of illness', so that Arthur Frank (1998) might pose the question, how can ill people become – without being patronised – the object of others people's solicitude? This is a practice that has, as one of its aims, the establishment of a positivity in illness (an illness *culture*), that emerges as complementary to health, not merely its shadow side.

The emergence of an illness culture has begun to alter the relationship between people and medicine. This is because stories of health care (sometimes critical, often trenchant) and pictures of coping with serious disease and its treatment contribute to new understandings about medicine, its possibilities and its limitations. Regarding the latter, it is possible to see self-reports about treatment and disease as emerging at the periphery of self-care that medical technologies create. Along with the growth of a consumer society, we might propose written and graphic accounts of illness as contributions to the kinds of changes sketched out above. And yet, this proposal is oversimplified if by this we mean that they have been instrumental only. This is not to undermine the role of patients' stories in the development of what has come to be called 'narrative medicine' (Charon, 2006), but for us to cast them in this role is to commit a sort of category mistake. Stories and pictures are not just instruments (in the sense of tools), nor are they mainly media channels along which ideas can be transmitted. This proposal historicizes them, turning them into steps, connections, or even reasons in a line of past events. Instead, I want to argue that, as 'works of illness', stories and pictures *are historical* (in the sense that Walter Benjamin used the term), in that they offer again and again the potential for critical re-appraisal at both individual and social level (Abbas, 1989).

Stories and pictures offer the possibility for re-imagining what it is to be ill in modern society; what, as an ill person, one has to offer and what one might expect to receive. How can that be? As representations they claim significance because they offer the chance to throw light on experiences refracted through them, as well as serving as a commentary on changes occurring in medicine and society. This does not preclude them being used to make claims about action toward change, but as aesthetic products their potential is not reducible to moral or political outcomes. What an aesthetic work makes possible is the reflection it invites by virtue of the way it takes up issues in the mundane world, including matters that came after its production. This is why a painting, a play or a poem written centuries ago, in another country and in another language, can resonate with audiences today. The expressive potential of such works is enhanced if they are used to make sense of later changes in the relationship of medicine to society. It could be said that this book is itself an example of such a way of 'making sensible', assembling a socio-cultural view of health and illness that underlines the semantic and aesthetic potential of the stories and pictures on which I base my argument.

Before beginning a detailed analysis of stories and pictures made by ill people – or what work these artefacts do – I want to raise questions about their acceptability. I mean this in the general sense of how the public, or the critics who mediate between producers and consumers of such works, respond to the idea that illness is something to be discussed, portrayed and opened to wider consideration. The acceptability of representations of illness is, in a rough and ready way, a useful measure of where matters concerning illness (and the sick as a group) stand in the scale of public concern. Of course, individual occasions of illness matter to each and every person in their turn, as do those of people near and dear to them. But the idea that illness might have some wider significance – is this a concern of recent origin, or perhaps of interest to so narrow a sector of society that it is still too fugitive to examine? What I mean here is not that the wider question of illness representation is too difficult to analyse, but that it is deemed of little importance compared to medical intervention. Telling about or showing illness is too transitory, so that dwelling on it detracts from the business of health care that is the mark of a robust economic and scientific approach to these matters. However, the response people have to stories and pictures about illness tells us something about the relationship of individuals to medicine, and hence to each other. This is important, as it sets these expressions of suffering, of healing and recovery, as well as dying, in the contexts which they ultimately reflect in making their meaning. There is, in that sense, a dialogic to the making of stories and pictures, involving give and take, acceptance and refusal, as well as the more analytical judgements made upon them.

Art for Illness's Sake

When the dance critic Arlene Croce wrote her non-review of Bill T. Jones's show in *The New Yorker* in 1994 she stirred up a hornet's nest of debate. It was (on her own admission) a non-review because Croce began the piece saying that she had not seen Jones's performance '*Still/Here*' and had no plans to do so. She gave as her reason that the show presented terminally ill people and talked about them. As such, Croce saw this as another example of 'victim art' that makes a claim upon its audience that is not intelligible as theatre. As a result, this made it impossible for her to criticise the performance from the perspective of art. What then, did she see this dance show as being? She said:

> If I understand '*Still/Here*' correctly, and I think I do – the publicity has been deafening – it is a kind of messianic travelling medicine show, designed to do some good for sufferers of fatal illnesses, both those in the cast and those thousand more who may be in the audience. (Croce, 1994: 54).

The problem for her was that, to review the show, she would have to be in the audience, where she would be forced to feel sorry for the dancers because of their status as terminally ill people. The charge she laid on them was that they used their victimhood as a strategy for eliciting something that went beyond compassion to 'induce, and even invite, a cozy kind of complicity' (1994: 55). This complicity works because the performers 'take sanctuary among the unwell', which together with the authority of theatre art, produces among some members of the audience a feeling of connection to what the performers are saying. These members of the audience are receptive to this message, says Croce, for the reason that, 'they are all co-religionists in the cult of the Self.' (1994: 56). Her response was to insist that she could not review someone whom she felt sorry for, or hopeless about.

The relevance of Croce's non-review for the present book is that many of the performers who participated in '*Still/Here*' were people with terminal illness, some with AIDS. As such they can be taken as representative of other seriously ill people who make art on the basis of their condition, while also being representative of other outgroups who make art from the margins. Her critique raised the wider question of the legitimacy of using illness as the basis for art, or rather of using art to fashion a statement about the social status of sick individuals or groups. It is not that illness cannot be the basis for 'great art', and Croce cites Schumann, Chopin and Keats as examples. Notably she says that 'painting pictures in their own blood' was, metaphorically speaking, what many such artists of the nineteenth century were doing. This is to be contrasted with the literal exemplification of suffering of which Croce accused AIDS victims, whom she saw as a 'pathetic lumping together, the individual absorbed by the group, the group by the disease' (1994: 59).

This piece was to remain an issue throughout Croce's career and would be returned to by others after her retirement. In a radio interview about Arlene

Croce, broadcast in 2005, the London based critic Jan Murray said of that review:

> One of the major forces behind Bill wanting to produce it was not the fact that he knew he was HIV positive and that his adored partner of 20 years had just died of AIDS...no, no, no, it was about working physically with feelings that are terribly hard to express otherwise, but also very hard to deal with on your own. So in the complete production, which was actually very moving and a lot of it was very joyous, you got clips of the various patients, all of whom had cancer (not all necessarily terminal) but working in movement groups, sometimes close-ups of faces. They were all unknown to the general public of course, and their voices were part of a running take, so you didn't know who was saying what, when. So you certainly didn't get any sort of confessions of desolation and horror from individuals. And of course the voices were cut through with music, and Bill's own beautiful company at that stage, all different sizes, shapes and colours, they did group dances with the odd solo that was representing aspects of illness, loss and death, but in the end it was very triumphant and positive about the possibilities of the human spirit. I know lots of people who were ill who saw that, certainly people who were HIV positive, nobody thought it was wallowing or it was misusing people who were dreadfully ill, because who were dancing but professional dancers, for goodness sake. I thought, what is she on about, this woman? (Australian Broadcasting Corporation, 2006).

As this commentary shows, Croce's non-review continues to raise a number of issues for anyone – including social scientists – interested in the articulation of illness as an aesthetic act. It is part of a social debate about the changing place of the sick in modern society, in relation both to the healthy and to other groups seen to be at the margins. Her piece treats us to a vision of the coerced, and ultimately rejecting healthy critic on the one hand, and the 'co-religionists' on the other. It is not difficult to deconstruct her argument to see the parallels of these groups with those appreciating 'great art' as compared with those seeking more immediate and easy gratification; those comprehending the ascetic distance required of art compared to those who enjoy bathing in the righteousness that (Croce says) comes from such works as 'Still/ Here'. Croce wrote from the perspective of an art critic and it is the transgression of her expertise by this and other shows like it that she most resented. This transgression led her to feel that her professional voice was silenced, though not just by the message of the performers. Almost more important, it was the feelings that these performers induced *in her* (a complicity of compassion) that she resisted by saying that it was 'forced' upon her. The problem would seem to be in the mixing of the realms of illness and art, of medicine and theatre, something that introduced for Croce an element that threatened the shape of artistic appreciation, as she knows and values it.

This localisation of the issue in this critic's response is important for the argument to be made in this book. This is not just because it raises issues about artistic levels or artistic merit; it also challenges ways in which people with serious illness might express their situation in 'artistic' ways or in venues associated with art. The former is not something to be passed over quickly here, because (as we shall see) people's views about what is to be considered 'art' are crucial in their judgements about the merits of work produced in the context of illness. One response to Croce's argument would be to ask her to examine further the feelings that shows such as '*Still/Here*' evoke *in her*, so that these might be entertained alongside other aesthetic judgements.

In her comment upon this non-review, the novelist and essayist Joyce Carol Oates made a similar point in saying that Croce would appear to be expressing, 'a revulsion for art with "power over the human conscience"' (1999: 71). She argued that even if art is too raw to be reviewed, shouldn't it be witnessed? This plea raises the question of what art is for. Is it for review? Is it for social change? Is it for therapy?

Oates claimed that it is unreasonable to expect the afflicted to transcend their fate in the name of art, and to demand that they do so in order to make audiences feel good is to insist on another sort of tyranny. She appears to respond here to the logical consequence of Croce's non-review that 'victims' should keep off the stage and maintain their suffering only as background to artistic work. In more general terms, this means a separation of art and illness, so that art retains its values and the sick know their place. The fact that they have a place already accorded to them is given in the very term 'victim art', a label 'so crude and reductive', says Oates, that it could only have been invented by someone unwilling to grant full humanity to those who have suffered injury, illness or injustice. This also raises the question as to whether the use of this term by the viewer makes it almost impossible to hear a message from the artist that cannot be reduced to the category of 'victim'.

However, there is another consequence to this separation of art and illness. This involves the silencing of *two* voices, one the voice of the afflicted artist and the other – equally important – the voice of the witness who would acknowledge the humanity expressed by the artwork. Lest we think that this applies only to minor artists or those who have little to say, consider the remarks made by the novelist John Updike when writing about his skin condition, psoriasis, and the effects it had on his life, 'It pains me to write these pages. They are humiliating – "scab-picking", to use a term sometimes levelled at modern autobiographical writers ' (1990: 44)

What is Updike's condition if it is not 'undiscussable'? What, if anything, makes or allows it to be discussable? These are questions that can only be answered once we admit the patient into the theatre, the aesthetic into the realm of illness. Asking these questions and debating them also raises issues about the rights and wrongs of illness and its treatment in society; about ways of representing disease; about the situation of those for whom relief from pain and suffering is difficult if not impossible and the situation of those who have to care for them. Equally important, it fuels the debate about how illness can and should be represented, about what cannot be represented and about the possible responses to these representations. Far from separating art and illness, there is much to be gained from allowing them to travel over each other's territory. I say 'travel' because it keeps open the options, does not reach for closure so that, for example, art is deemed 'good for illness' or equally that illness is necessarily thought to be 'good for art'. I am acknowledging here what others have already pointed out about Croce's piece on Bill T. Jones; that it reflects a breakdown in the categories between illness, art and science, indeed in the locus of the voice of authority where disease and its treatment is concerned (Diedrich, 2007). This can result in difficulty in the apprehension of meaning, and in accompanying attempts to restore the status quo (as Croce tried to do). What it offers subsequently – now – is the possibility of exploring this *dedifferentiation* of meanings of illness to describe how representation is being re-made with regard to new forms (or old forms in new places) and the relationship of people to medicine.

If Croce's non-review aims at preserving art from illness – or more precisely, from the sick – then the commentaries of Grover (1989) and of Crimp (1992) were aimed at saving the sick from the ministrations of art. Both of these authors were critical of a photography exhibition, "*Pictures of People*" (accompanying booklet, Nixon, 1988), presented at the Museum of Modern Art in New York. The exhibition showed a series of portraits of people, some with AIDS, taken by the photographer Nicholas Nixon. Crimp noted that the exhibition was well-received and he quotes from generous reviews testifying to the way in which the viewer might feel 'both vulnerable and privileged to share the life and (impending) death of a few individuals' (Atkins, quoted in Crimp, 1992: 117); and that with the gradual disappearance of the subjects' self-consciousness, 'the camera seems to become invisible, and consequently there is almost no boundary between the image and ourselves' (Grundberg, quoted in Crimp, 1992: 117). Crimp was critical of these portraits on the grounds that they presented people with AIDS in such a way as to maintain a sense of otherness under the guise of understanding. This understanding is an achievement of the way in which they were photographed. By showing them ravaged and disfigured, alone and desexualised, they are sequestered in ways that in previous years would only be possible by physical isolation. This portrayal is made possible by a focus upon the personal and the private, excluding the public (the contextual) issues that give people with AIDS a history, a locus, a biography. This exclusion of context was the focus for protest by the New York AIDS activist group ACT UP, who staged a protest in the gallery. Their demand was for the visibility of people with AIDS who are 'vibrant, angry, loving, sexy, beautiful, acting up and fighting back' (quoted in Grover, 1989: 14).

From one perspective this reveals how portraiture can render the people portrayed as having no identity other than as victims of AIDS, while also providing the public with the 'face of AIDS' that gave tangible form to a relatively new and frightening disease (Gilman, 1995). As Crimp noted, the best that such images can do is to 'elicit pity, and pity is not solidarity' (1992: 126). There is a demand then, that afflicted people create their own images but, as Crimp argues, this means not taking 'truer' pictures (if that were possible) but relating activism about AIDS to the condition of the image construction as a representation. In a similar vein, it has been suggested that the use of the photographic close-up that Nixon employed in some of these pictures – perhaps as dramatic revelations – are in the end repellent (Ogdon, 2001). This response comes from the fact that people do not see these minutiae in everyday relationships, so that to present them in this way is to reduce the subject, in what might be seen as the search for the 'unfathomable Thing' that is at the base of being a person with AIDS. Somehow, presenting the detail of the body of the person with AIDS, says Ogdon, subverts the representation that would acknowledge and even celebrate (if that is possible) their social situation.

Taking this line reminds us that photography is both an act of presentation and representation, though unlike Ogdon I would not set these two positions against one another. The idea of 'presenting' should not be reduced to a search for the Real, any more than 'representing' should be elevated to a pursuit of the socially significant. The aims and values of representation and the techniques and materials of presentation are essential to the arguments I shall make about how affected individuals show others what illness means.

In the case of the Nixon exhibition, the fact that it was shown at MOMA made a claim about the artistic merit of the pictures, about the skills of the photographer and about the possible responses of the viewer. What work does 'art' do to enable a response by the viewer to such photographs? In the introduction to the book accompanying the *Pictures of People* exhibition (Nixon, 1988), Peter Galassi compares Nixon's work to that of Diane Arbus, who he said, 'cut through the public scene to the private person and made herself emotionally present in her work' (Galassi, 1988: 27). Far from reading such comments in a positive light, Grover (1989), in a trenchant critique, points out that references to the photographer's sensibility, to his skill in encouraging the sitter to hold nothing back, to his surrogate witnessing of pain all point to the understanding of the portrayals as works of the artist. The assembly of a series of such portraits also serves to do something very important, which is to lead the viewer to search for the general, the essence inhabiting the faces of all who are pictured. What this encourages in the viewer (at least, the critic) is the sense of finding something about humanity, assumed to be somehow inside the viewer (photographer). This is something that speaks to a belief 'that art is about "timeless realities", "enduring values", "the human condition", and thence to viewers who prefer wispy abstractions to the historical and specific' (Grover, 1989). The accusation is that 'art' – at least of this kind – does not help the situation of people with AIDS: it positively hinders it.

This example of a conflict over visual representation is a useful comparison to make with the debate over performance art, both concerning the situation of people with AIDS. On the one hand, Croce strives to preserve art at the expense of hearing the voice of afflicted people. On the other hand, Crimp and Grover seek to empower afflicted people by freeing them from the representations of the photographer/artist, and of the media. At a superficial level there is a sense that art and illness do not mix, that the values of art – the general essences that stem from its transcendent qualities – cannot serve the needs of ill people.

The question of whether art (with a capital 'A') should be used to promote the needs of ill people is not the main concern of this book. Nor is my concern the effects of the performer/artist's illness upon art in general, as with the consequences of personal illness upon an artist's work. Instead, the interesting point about these two debates is that they bear upon the way that ideas of illness are being re-fashioned, and the way that the relationship of illness to health is being worked out through these notions. However, these debates are not just about ideas – in the sense of arguments – but are also about ways of making, showing, and consuming tangible works. The questions that press forward are about the kinds of works produced, under what conditions, made by whom and with what claims to authenticity and legitimacy. They are also about the ways in which illness is made up and shown forth in these various genres and arenas, so that the practices that are deemed to be 'art' (not necessarily fine art or high art) deserve attention. This is important if we are to find out what can be said about illness through these works that cannot easily be said in another way. Perhaps we should replace the word 'said' with the word 'shown'. Is this something to do with the ill person's 'self', as Croce says, in her condemnation of *'Still/Here?* Or is it something concerning the social context of illness, its treatment and the relationship of the sick to the healthy?

Stories of Illness: 'pathography' as social science

The risks of speaking out as an ill person – or on behalf of the afflicted – are not limited to those inhabiting the world of art. In the social sciences the emergence of a body of work that can broadly be called the study of 'illness narratives' has attracted critical attention from scholars wanting to draw lines between art and science. The number of books written by sufferers describing their disease, but especially serious diseases like cancer, seems to have grown over the last quarter century. This has extended into newspaper reports by individuals who have given blow-by-blow accounts of their symptoms, their treatment and the effects that this has had upon their life and the lives of those around them. At one level, these stories concern encounters with medicine and the ups and downs of treatments that are more or less successful in halting disease. At another level, each is a personal narrative of the way that the person has coped with the life-changes consequent upon the diagnosis, and the likelihood of leading life in the shadow of what has happened to them (Couser, 1997; Frank, 1995). The accounts that have appeared in the popular media and books have been considered to be journalistic pieces, albeit ones that seem to be creating a new genre, or answering what might be a previously unmet need among the public to know about illness experience (Greenslade, 1997). The question here is perhaps the relationship between the need to tell and the need to know, so that some might think that we have moved into a society that has an almost 'unhealthy' interest in ill health, if that is possible.

Interestingly, it was Joyce Carol Oates (the critic of Croce), who wrote about what she saw as biographers' unfortunate focus upon the misfortunes of their subjects. Instead of artists drawing attention to their own plight, this accusation is aimed at commentators who attempt an understanding of art in terms of the pathologies of their subjects, including their illnesses. Oates (1988) saw this as a symptom of a wider cultural pathology, where an understanding of art is reduced to the shortcomings of the self. However, others have seen this form of writing – albeit in autobiographic form – as a sign of cultural health. That health comes from a much needed acknowledgement of our condition as embodied selves, an embodiment that has, in relation to illness, so far been a 'literary no man's land' (Couser, 1991). It has been claimed that telling about one's illness provides both a model for analytic writing about the body (a 'communicative body') and an opportunity for writer and reader together to be brought into a new relationship to each other (a 'lived ethics of bodies'), (Frank, 1997). Where Oates was criticising the searching out of misfortune as a way of explaining a life, writers of illness narratives would seem to be searching out a life after misfortunes that have been thrust upon them. Perhaps more important for the present discussion, where Oates was concerned about the content of such stories, people like Frank and Couser seem to be pointing to them as doing a particular kind of work in the course of shaping their message.

If this kind of work – this way of telling – is missing from the story, then autobiographies of illness would hardly be art, though one doubts if many are written with that aspiration (which means, arguably, that some do achieve this status). Why care whether they are art or not? Because if they are not art then the question arises – as we shall see below – are they documents, or science, if we mean by this the social kind? As Clarke aptly put it, it 'is not that griping can't be artful, but rather we shouldn't assume that all memoir is artful when it gripes.' (1999: B9). The key issue dividing the merely confessional from the artistic is, in his view, the ways that the author/artist finds to represent life's difficulties, what she does to shape it. This shaping is a matter of drawing upon and appealing to aesthetic sensibilities, matters that exercise an ascetic distance so that sentimentality and vitriol are excluded from the account. In the end it is not the truth of the story that matters, 'but how the author makes a story *seem* true (Clarke, 1999: B9, emphasis in original).

These comments are reminiscent of Croce's critique, and once again alert us to the fact that accounts of illness, as well as representations made or performed on behalf of illness, are created in a postmodern climate where the confessional mode encourages all kinds of self-revelation (Furedi, 2004). In radio interviews, on television, and in print people are given space to air their stories within media frames that invite listeners, viewers and readers to identify with the experiences of the person concerned. As a result, the relationship produced is less one of people *in* their world, a conjunction with the historical moment, but one of people's selves *as* their world, where the totalising of similar experience adds nothing to its revelation, to the potential for its understanding.

This is the danger risked by all who today write the story of their illness, who make pictures on behalf of it or otherwise create works inspired by it. One answer is to eschew entirely the details of one's own illness experience (of one's *self*) in order to focus upon the disease itself, or to adopt (even if only partially) a framework of abstraction that make it possible to keep a distance in order that illness is rendered sensible to others. This involves more than sense: it also involves a sensibility that is accorded to the reader for whom distance from personal material is thereby guaranteed. A good example of this is Susan Sontag's (1978) book *'Illness as Metaphor'*, written after her experience of treatment for breast cancer. This book was an instant success, not least with social scientists, who saw it as providing a further inroad into the biological hegemony of disease. It fitted with the idea that illness is 'socially constructed', in particular with the claim that language shapes our understanding of the world and that it is wielded inequitably by different social groups. It seemed to take some time before these commentators realised that Sontag was arguing for the *removal* of the cultural baggage of metaphor from cancer, so as to benefit those suffering from the disease. She did this – she said later – for practical reasons, to deprive 'cancer' of its meanings. These meanings give it the power to signify, powers that rebound on its sufferers in the frightening tropes that, as harmless adjectives attaching to the world when one is healthy, re-surface to wound when the person is diagnosed with cancer. Most relevant for our concerns here is what Sontag said about her aim in writing her book:

> I didn't think it would be useful – and I wanted to be useful – to tell one more story in the first person of how someone learned that she or he had cancer, wept, struggled, was comforted, suffered, took courage, … though mine was also that story. A narrative, it seemed to me, would be less useful than an idea. (Sontag, 1991: 98).

In saying this, Sontag was not criticising the first-person story as such, but saying that she had the skills to fashion an instrument to dissolve metaphor, to go, in her terms, 'against interpretation'. This instrument might be regarded as an artefact, artfully constructed so as to provide a meaningful purchase on cancer and how it might be borne and understood. It serves best as a weapon to counter the prejudices that surround disease, a plank in the platform built by activists trying to forge a better deal for cancer sufferers and their treatment. In that sense a book about an idea – as an instrument – has a generality, an application to something else that one wishes to change. This is in contrast to a story about one's illness that is not instrumental in quite this way, because it is not general, is not applicable in the same sense. A story that someone tells about his or her life might become, in its extrapolation, a moral tale, but in the telling its power lies in its origin as well as in its application. For the moment it is enough to say that stories 'in the first person', whether or not they are artful, work in a different way to the presentation of 'an idea'. And in doing that they risk being accused of other shortcomings in addition or in place of the charge that they are not art. This charge is that they are 'bad science'.

The idea of bad science is linked to the weakening of methodology, those procedures that are established in order that investigators can share the view that certain things happened because of what was done to bring them about. In a sense, methods are instruments for the entertainment of ideas, which they focus on their objects of inquiry. In respect of illness as a topic for the sociology of medicine, a weakening of method can be linked to an erosion of the distance between observer and object, and the associated reversal of the influence between the two. The world shapes selves: selves do not ('should not') shape the world. It has been said that the presentation of illness narratives as important sources of data in the field of illness experience commits both of these offences against good science.

Atkinson and Silverman (1997), both sociologists, have argued that the study of illness narratives has privileged these stories in ways that are not justified. The kernel of their argument is that stories of illness – presented as data – participate in an error that preserves the self over against the social world. Taking the author's standpoint on the world, these narratives do not sufficiently comprehend the social context (the other voices) that constitute the experience that the narrator takes as her or his own. Stemming from a Romantic agenda, which sets self apart from the world and privileges the former, this program of work has as its twin aims the celebration of the subject and the commitment to therapeutic practice. This therapeutic practice is worked through in the redemptive possibilities of narrative itself, so that the act of story telling is reconstitutive of self, a self whose harmony and coherence is basic to the idea of survival and recovery from serious illness. What appears to follow from this is that the study of autobiographical accounts might be assumed to allow access to what Atkinson (1997) called 'a realm of hyperauthenticity', a truth only to be tested against the author's experience, the writer's feelings.

This view resonates with the idea of a confessional society, such that the use of face-to-face interviews might be thought to provide deeper or more truthful accounts of life experience. Instead – as a good scientist would – of holding firm to method, authors who traffic in autobiographies of illness risk invoking a neo-Romantic inner self, one whose special journey into and out of suffering somehow entitles them to report back to the healthy on a land where they, and a few others, have travelled and made the journey back. Their experience (if not their survival) is their authority, and the celebration of the overcoming of their troubles a sufficient proof of the significance of their lives. The point at which readers enter into this celebration – similar to what Croce called a 'cozy kind of complicity' – creates what Atkinson and Silverman (drawing upon the novelist Milan Kundera) referred to as '*homo sentimentalis*'. This is a cultural idea of someone who is 'not to be defined as a man with feelings (for we all have feelings), but as a man who has raised feelings to a category of value' (Kundera, quoted in Atkinson and Silverman, 1997: 321). Pointing up the redundancy of criticisms of the Romantic self – its supposed isolation, integrity and truth – these critics highlight the pointlessness of a search for authenticity when the very idea is under question. This false search is to be contrasted with what these authors term 'the realities of everyday professional or social-science practice.' Only by holding on to these 'realities' will (sociologists) keep themselves from the perils of the self-revealing speaking subject, and (and this is not to be underestimated) protect themselves from the inevitable *distaste* that follows encounters with such kitsch as the video diary.

One way to understand this debate is to draw upon a view of modernism, such as provided by Habermas (1996), who described the emergence of three autonomous spheres – art, justice and science – as 'magnificent onesidednesses' (p. 328) that, once separated from the everyday world, undermine the truth claims of local experience. The result of this has been to produce a 'fragmented consciousness' of the everyday that further allows these three moments of reason to colonize the lifeworld. It is against this background, and along what Habermas calls the seams between system and lifeworld, that resistance and protest occur. Related to questions of illness, it is easy to make an argument for the appearance of works of illness as forms of protest against the authority of scientific medicine, the latter seen as an aesthetic of good taste and a morality grounded upon orthodox heterosexuality. Stories and pictures protest not only at the incursions of unmediated spheres of expertise (e.g. of medicine) but also at the fragmentation and dismissal of local practices and knowledge grounded in the everyday.

In turn, those who criticise works of illness on the grounds of 'bad taste', 'romanticism' or even 'revolution' respond in their own terms to forms of protest about how ill people are treated or viewed by others. However, this idea of spheres that include, exclude and distil out leaves the kinds of works we have been considering as too passive, as too reactionary. It is as if, once having told their story or made their picture, works become subject to conventions that rule them in or out of the worlds of art or science. However, it is important to note that part of this procedure is premised upon each sphere having a limited understanding of the terms of the others. For example, at the end of a study of how astronomers use aesthetic judgements in the course of their work – but do not acknowledge this – it has been said:

> Scientists are unlikely to understand their ordinary practice as deeply 'aesthetic' in orientation, since this would require a profound change not only in their understanding of aesthetics, but *in the modern conception as well.* (Lynch and Edgerton, 1988: 214, emphasis added).

Such a change in conception would be demanded of social scientists too, which is precisely what is argued by those working with stories in the realm of response to medical treatment. This puts in question whether the issue of authenticity should be treated as one of versions made by ill people compared to those made by doctors or social scientists. It should, instead, be about the authenticity of the person in relation to their illness experience. Truth then is not about the 'true self', but the truth that is spoken to illness. Citing Arthur Frank, whose work was one focus for Atkinson's critique, Bochner raised the options for sociology in relation to encouraging individual sufferers to speak and be heard. Of special note, I think, is an almost simple case he makes for authenticity being viewed not in terms of its possibility, but in terms of an ideal to which we might aspire. This, then, is not an empirical question but an ethical one. The words that Bochner uses are: 'whether the ideal of authenticity is good and useful'. Continuing, he says, shouldn't 'a good sociology oppose suffering, promote healing, and give agency to marginalized identities? (Bochner, 2001: 147). The notion of 'goodness' springs from quite a different place to the concerns of Atkinson and Silverman, for whom the practical aims of work with and for people who tell stories of illness is secondary. Goodness is certainly an ethical concern, but one so broad in this context as to be easy to pass over.

In defence of his own position, Frank (2000a) is adamant in his agreement with Atkinson's perception of his (Frank's) standpoint in ethics being a qualitatively different one to that of empiricist sociology. He rejects methodological integrity as the basis for his work, stressing that ethical principles command a different approach to story telling. These principles are not reducible to some interior self but take their meaning from the practice of stories being told, and listened to by others. It is what happens in the hearing of the story, the acknowledgment and the affirmation of experience, that authenticity can be achieved. From this perspective authenticity is more a judgement about an open-ended meeting of people, not a quality to be unearthed from an interior self. Stories, Frank says, address the problem of how we can live life differently, showing in their form and content an alternative way of being, where that being matters because, in part, it is about living with serious illness. Interestingly, he uses as an explanatory device the common reversible image of the duck-rabbit, saying that one has to engage with the figure until the reverse image appears. Listening to stories – entertaining the possibility that they might show you something new – means attending for long enough to participate in their shape and form. From this position, working with people's stories must always be about engagement rather than distance.

What are we to make of this? If one works within the sociological frame then this debate is about the kind of sociology that one should pursue. However, this is not the frame that I wish to put up at this point. At the risk of skimming over important methodological issues, I would rather treat this debate as another example of the difficult and shifting ground that works of illness occupy, whether they are autobiographical accounts, dance performances or photographs. In this exchange between social scientists, the accusations are not about whether stories about illness 'are art', but whether they constitute 'good science'. There are some quite distinct issues here, regarding the status of the concept of self and the concern with transparency in methodological techniques. But there are some common issues too, relating to the perceived elevation of self in autobiographical writing. This concerns the movement toward a person's own experience as the basis for determining significance and value, with the concomitant risk of eroding the institutionalised guides for determining independently whether the work produced is 'good art' or, in another context, 'good science'. The valuation of the person's point of view is indeed part of the interview society, in which the confessional has become one of the bread and butter constituents of the Internet, television and the print media. The other side of the confessional is where other people's tragedies become a spectacle for the infotainment of the viewer/reader. Somehow, whenever people write about their illness, or portray its effects in other ways, they will no doubt wish to distinguish it from the 'kitsch' of video-diary culture. And, as everyday critics, would we not wish to entertain the possibility that works are made that transcend mere griping and self-serving sentimentality? Arguably, it trivialises people's illness stories to refer to them as 'confessionals' or to mock them as 'hyperauthentic'

(Bochner, 2001: 147), and that to do so is to miss much of what they have to teach.

The further point is that we might also miss *how* they teach us. This is important because the way in which stories and other works bring about their effects is constitutive of the orientation we take to illness, to the suffering person in particular and to the sick in general. The efforts that ill people make to fashion their experiences into a tangible form might or might not be successful, but to understand how they succeed or fail in this regard is to throw light on the fabrication of illness in the modern age.

Before pursuing this point further, it is worth noting that some of the most influential accounts of illness have been written by people able to speak with the voices of various realms of knowledge when describing their own illness. In a way this gives an extra turn to the issue of authenticity, in that the producer and commentator on the story are the same person. For example, Arthur Frank has written the story of his illness in '*At the Will of the Body*', in which he says, 'But I do not write as any kind of expert; I present myself only as a fellow sufferer, trying to make sense of my own illness.' (1991: 5). In subsequent publications (1995, 2004) he has developed a sociological position in which he uses his story as an exemplar of the possibilities of story telling by other people. (This is one of the positions criticised by Atkinson and Silverman.) I do not mean that Frank projects his story on to others, but that he finds it (or aspects of it) being reflected back to him in the stories told by fellow sufferers.

One of the difficulties here is that autobiographical statements that bear upon illness experience are not appropriate for third party checking because they are not matters of fact, nor are their claims subject to falsification. The fears and delights that are described by an author about his or her illness and its relief are better considered to be *avowals* rather than statements of fact (Shotter, 1981). As such, they are matters to be accepted or refused, witnessed or ignored, acknowledged or doubted, but not tested empirically. As readers of published accounts, we need to be persuaded that such and such was the case, that it was just this way, that what is being described has the *semblance* of truth. And there is one further thing – we need to be persuaded (if we approach the question of illness from any other than a personal basis) that the account matters. This question, concerning significance, seemingly refers to issues that are beyond the immediacy of the description given, whether they are matters of content or of form or of history. Failure to persuade on these counts can leave the illness story as just one more account, but not a 'telling narrative' that promotes political action, galvanises support, elaborates theory or elicits an aesthetic response.

Where a story fails on all these counts then its power to influence is likely to be limited to the personal. This is not a failure to be a story – or to be useful to individual readers – but if considered in the context of art or science or letters then it is likely to be marked by the shortcomings stemming from the particular benchmarks applied to it. This seems to be the basis of the charges laid by Croce in the realm of art, and by Atkinson and Silverman in the realm of science as to what people in different circumstances have shown and told about their illnesses. I am not trying here to rescue these performances and stories – I am not in a position to do so. Rather, I am pointing to the idea that they have a kind of history of their own, as works that aspire – more or less – to be simultaneously what they are and yet more than what they are. And we should remember that the fate of works of whatever kind extends to their being appraised in contexts different from the ones for which they were intended, so that those created for therapeutic/political reasons can become data for social science, or can be displayed in a gallery for the interest and pleasure of visitors. In these cases other criteria will likely be applied to the works and as a consequence they will be treated differently. For example, whatever makes a 'good story' does not finish once it is written but continues in the way it is received and reviewed.

I said above that significance 'seemingly' refers to issues beyond the work, and I hold to the idea that stories, pictures and performances about illness are meaningful in terms of realms of discourse applied to them. However, there is a sense in which some stories and art works – like a good case study – create and sustain the reader/viewer's engagement in a way that evokes its own significance. At this point I want to make this claim in order to underline the idea that what matters is that stories of illness should *seem* true, that they should have the *semblance* of truth. This is not to assert that they are false any more than to say that they are true. That option is denied us once we give up the idea that such stories are repositories of facts or even of memory traces; and once we give up the idea that they are descriptive of some interior self, or that they comprise the authentic voice of the writer. Instead, there is something about the effective establishment of the 'semblance of truth', where that semblance is held to matter in some important way. Much of the remainder of this book is an exploration of how this happens and its implications for understanding what we mean by 'illness' (and also 'health') as a consequence.

Increasingly, in this section, I have referred to stories along with 'other works' and in doing so tipped my hand to show that these things are products that are given shape by their creators. This shape is yet another broad way of saying that they are fabricated, that they share with artworks the important criterion of semblance as key to conveying significance about what it means to be seriously ill, to undergo treatment, to recover, or to face the prospect of dying. All these are matters to do with ways of living, so that there is an ethical dimension to all of this, something made explicit by writers such as Bochner and Frank in their defence of a position that is not science (in the sense of an empiricism) and, one supposes, not art. Story telling for them is a redemptive practice, and being so directs our attention to something like Foucault's (1980) idea of 'problematising life as a work of freedom'. But we have seen that it is not just freedom that is at issue here, but matters of taste and distaste, which judgement comes into play when things are brought out from the realm of the sick into the world of the healthy. These are matters of aesthetic judgment, to which I will turn in the next section.

Writing and Performing Illness: aesthetic or aestheticist?

The insistence that stories of illness are ethical in principle – or that they are told and heard within an ethical frame – is important for considering their status. For Frank (2000b) the question of ethics is determinable in the way that the authors of such stories demonstrate that they became who they are by making choices; that things could have been otherwise. These choices are not just about the self, but concern how to act in the face of events arising from one's illness or that of another person. These events presume that the world of the ill is not an isolated world, but one touched by the everyday, by the social and historical. An illness biography, then, is a demonstration of which choices were made and why, of what was done in the light of circumstance, others' actions, and one's own feelings.

How these things bear upon the author then becomes the issue when critics wish to determine the status of the account. Should it appear (for whatever reason) that the author/performer privileges their subjectivity in whatever way, then the work is seen to fall short, somehow exposing the author/performer in particular ways. On the one hand, the person is seen to be making an unwarranted moral claim regarding their fate or social circumstance (e.g. Croce's [1994] reaction to being made to feel sorry by people presenting themselves as 'dissed blacks, abused women, disenfranchised homosexuals'). This operates at what we might call a mundane level. On the other hand, the author/performer appears to be making a claim of a different kind, about their judgemental ability or rather, their special taste. This is an expressive claim, value laden but carrying implications of superior knowledge or experience. It is the kind of claim that

| 33

might be forthcoming from those with serious illness who have travelled near to death and returned to share their special knowledge with others.

Here, no doubt, is one source of the charge of Romanticism laid against the illness biographers. They are able to affect an air of superior knowledge, and somehow (wrongly? unfairly?) benefit from being reflected in the light of their own story, or else that of other people's stories that they interpret. The self that is elevated can be said to claim the status of an arbiter of taste as a result of the person's experiences. It is, in one sense, an aesthetic self that emerges, not least because the experiences in question are to do with suffering and death. To the extent that this is presented as or seen to be a brush with the sublime, then that is sufficient to promote further the idea that the author/performer is making a claim to exercise aesthetic judgements. That this 'brush' might be sufficient for all who are touched by it to make such a claim is suggested by the idea that:

> Artists with AIDS live in a world where artistic and moral concerns have become contiguous, where matters of style are momentous because all speaking out about oneself is a matter of painting on the broad canvas of life and death and history. (Chandler, 1991: 63)

This suggestion appears to assimilate the world to the self, or at least to be saying that the contiguity of art and illness somehow guarantees insights in this field, a view that is arguably too ambitious.

Instead of this, I want to bring forward the essential but sometimes occluded side of accusations about the kind of works we are considering. Croce's piece is well known because of her outspokenness about this aspect. When it comes to the 'bad science' critiques, the use of the words 'Romantic' and 'privilege' in respect of the work are key to the fact that only half of what is being criticised is the product; the other half is the author. The attempt is to locate the error in the actions of the authors/performers concerned. The charge is, in blunt terms, that of being 'aestheticist' in one's professional life, operating a kind of 'flabby' aestheticism (Osborne, 1997). This is to be contrasted with being aesthetic, in the sense of employing an ethic in order to problematise 'ordinary' experience and conduct one's life in terms consistent with this modality.

Aesthetic work held to be of critical value always presupposes *asceticism*, which is to say a distance between the producer and the work. This is important if the product is to sustain itself as a commentary on the world, rather than be absorbed back into it. This distance reflects a commitment to the necessities of the action field where the constraints are freely chosen, making possible a kind of exemplary freedom (Osborne, 1998: 117). This is the basis of the idea that the aesthetic is ethical, that in the context of illness the way of dealing with fate is by problematising life rather than fashioning forms of escapism and self-indulgence. The freedom so created refers also to matters of public morality, concerning issues surrounding the ways that the sick are expected to live, expectations fashioned both inside and outside of medicine. The twin pressures of public morality and private fate are summary terms for the fields of constraint in which persons must work when responding to disease. As a way of legitimising one's suffering and establishing one's normality in spite of illness, it has been said that public morality has to be merged with private fate (Gerhardt, 1989: 214). This is an accurate view of events seen from the perspective of the need to disavow the stigma of illness, but this assumes that the answer to illness is adjustment (conformity) not problematisation involving testimony and witness.

The ideas of 'aestheticism' and 'the aesthetic' need, however, to be seen in their historical context. A concern with aestheticism is both a modernist and a postmodern one. The fact that Romanticism can today be levelled as an accusation is because of the part it played in de-historicising the link between alienation and creativity, and in removing the realm of art from the everyday world. These two moments together produced the conditions under which marginal individuals were first the objects of fascination for artists and then became the source of their own special creativity (Bowler, 1997). It is as if the majority found in the alterity of marginal persons some aspect of their own artistic inclination, much as colonizers were doing with pre-literate peoples in the far corners of the world (Taussig, 1993). (Indeed, the idea of colonization of the patient's body by medicine in the course of treatment has been referred to directly by authors such as Arthur Frank in his writings and by artists such as Jo Spence in commentaries about her photographs.) We can see here a parallel with an interest in the sick, so that it is precisely on these grounds that Grover accused the MOMA gallery of displaying photographs that elevated the photographer over the person with AIDS, by effectively setting forth Nixon's concerns in the images of the individuals depicted.

Lyotard (1984) argued that the experience of serious illness can be perceived as an experience so immense or powerful that it can only be considered 'without reason'. By this he meant that no concept adequately binds the phenomenon. One has only to think of pain, suffering and the fear of death to see that serious illness, with its dissolution of bodily integrity, is a field ripe for the making of such images. Works of illness, conceived in this way, conform to Lyotard's conviction that the aesthetic is a way of bearing witness to the world. But this itself presupposes that disinterestedness – that ascetic distance – which has already been mentioned. The subject matter of works of illness cannot in itself guarantee anything about their eventual status, as we have already seen. Indeed, the very idea of presenting objects that fail to match concepts is to risk being accused, at the least, of woolly thinking, and worse still, of Romanticism.

What remains to be determined is what is it about such works that make them successful, or relevant or even solicitous? This is not to apply aesthetics to illness as if it could enlighten us about subjects like pain and suffering, but to engage with the idea that there is a different way of fashioning experience, of presenting meaning, of rendering life's conundrums somehow graspable. This is perhaps inconsistent with Osborne's (1997) insistence that sociologists (to whom his remarks are addressed) need to look at core aesthetic practices first, before extending these type-cases to other examples. His insistence comes, I think, from the motive to avoid being aetheticist at all costs, to avoid intellectualising about aesthetics, or thinking that one can somehow apply aesthetic principles in chosen fields of social research.

However, if aesthetics is an ethic that transforms the world, attaining, in the course of this, autonomy of practice and existence – a kind of freedom – then dissecting where and how that ethic operates in works of illness is a potentially valuable exercise. While ideas about illness are shaped by medicine and by discourses of risk, the technological innovations that make survival possible create spaces in people's lives. By spaces I do not mean neutral clearings, well lit and undemanding, but chasms of doubt and relief, anxiety and hope that can merge into times of impenetrable, cloaking fear. To take one simple example – supplied as an adjunct to the rehearsal of a play about breast cancer, '*Handle with Care*' – a woman tells of being in the car with her husband, after a radiation oncologist has informed her that her longest surviving patient with metastatic disease lived for 23 years. The woman says:

> And there it was – long distance hope. I was thrilled. I told my husband during the drive home. 'Twenty-three years', I said. 'Can you believe it?' 'Of course', he replied with that I-told-you-so-look of smugness. Well, I lost it! I wanted to pull the car over and whack him one. I was livid because he was dismissing my reality, my fear, my agony. Sure – one patient lived for 23 years, and maybe I will too. The fact that one did opened up a world of possibilities. But it's a long shot and it's the not knowing, and being all too aware of the statistics that makes this disease hell. And I've learned to live with this hell and even become brilliant at it at times –and I didn't want him minimizing all that with his glib, 'Of course'. (Gray, Sinding, Ivonoffski, Fitch, Hampson and Greenberg, (2000: 140).

This quote is introduced as a story that became part of the play, thus becoming a refractive piece speaking to the audience's views about the disease. I cite it here because it illustrates nicely this notion of spaces created by medical help, spaces that open up in the everyday world of the people concerned, to which they respond in a variety of ways. All advances in medicine that impinge on people through technology and information create potentials where, in Lyotard's terms, the imagination fails to present an object which might, if only in principle, come to match a concept (Osborne, 1997: 133). It does not follow that people must make art out of their anxieties. (In the case cited above, we can only wonder what the woman means when she says she has become 'brilliant' at living with her personal hell.) Whether people do or do not make art, their response to illnesses that are manageable but not curable shapes both their relationship to medicine and to society itself.

The consideration of how people shape their experience of illness for others – and for themselves – is an important task for anyone interested in ideas about illness in the modern world. Whether those efforts – what I am calling *works of illness* – are worthy of being called 'art' is really another matter. But if they can be understood in terms of aesthetic practice – of an ethic that problematises the person's situation as a work of freedom – then this is very much a concern for those wanting to examine changing meanings of health and illness. Even though the status of many such works as 'art objects' is by the way, this does not rule out the influence that such a designation might have on their influence more generally. In the case of the play, '*Handle with Care*', the theatrical context invited a closeness of engagement that the authors see as an 'ecological view of ethics', one containing risk, danger and vulnerability. How this closeness squares with the disinterestedness that Osborne holds as vital to the ascetic attitude is something for us to discuss later on. At this point, his comment that 'the production of works of art, as an aspiration, takes the form of a practical reflection on the possibility of autonomy' (1998: 110) can make a starting point for examining the ways in which ill people have tried to fashion a kind of freedom for themselves and for others.

Towards an 'aethestics of illness'

The following quotation might stand as a caution to those wanting to write about aesthetics, whether in the context of health or otherwise.

> Those who say that they are artists or who claim to be using artistic
> principles in their work, and – worse – those who intellectualize about
> such principles: these are always the most embarrassing kinds of people.
> (Osborne, 1998: 122)

The first two charges I can easily avoid; I am not an artist and I do not use
artistic principles in my work. The danger, it seems, is in writing about
aesthetic practices as employed by ill people wanting to make a statement
about their own or other people's situations. One would hope to avoid the
more serious charge of 'intellectualizing about such principles', which might
result from elevating them to a position not warranted by the facts. In spite
of that, Osborne's concern that one should not be 'aestheticist' is still risked
where an examination of narratives or portrayals might aestheticise the
author/artist. This after all, is the accusation made by Sontag (and repeated in
a different context by Atkinson and Silverman) concerning the
romanticisation of the sick. In another context – that of social theory –
Osborne accuses Maffesoli of aestheticising people in terms of his concept of
neo-tribes (Maffesoli, 1991), in order to take a 'detached pleasure in their
somewhat laughable kitsch' (Osborne, 1997: 139). Aestheticisation is a way of
patronising people, where as a parallel outcome, the person conferring the
judgment draws attention to his or her sophisticated taste.

How to avoid this? In my view the aim of exploring 'works of illness' is
not to apply aesthetic principles to the sick, but to explore how illness
provides an arena for making artefacts that express something of that world.
This opens up the possibility – though not the certainty – that these works
can be understood as deriving their significance from the deployment of an
ethic of freedom, realised in terms of aesthetic practice. This is not to try to
determine 'works of illness' to be 'works of art' as judged in the public
sphere. Whether stories or paintings made by ill people are 'art with a capital
A' is really of secondary concern here, though should others label them in
this way then this will matter, and we should want to know how it affects
their significance in understanding health.

What seems to me of importance is to address squarely why and how ill
people might want to use artistic portrayal as the means to say important
things about their experience and their situation. What can one say or show
in this way that is not said more directly or more clearly from a medical,
scientific or documentary perspective? To answer this question one needs to
examine in detail the way that such works 'do their job', both in the mode of
presentation and in the apparent response that they call out in other people.
This project does not depend, as I have said above, on determining stories

and pictures as products removed from the everyday world of usefulness. Ill people continue to live in a world where social ethics relating to conduct as a patient or carer continue to operate and to which they are likely to subscribe. The aesthetic is not a totalising realm that replaces these, but is rather a domain opened up when these other spheres are problematised (Hunter, 1992). Coupled with this point, nor should the aesthetic be thought of as a way of harmonising or bringing together these various realms in some artistic/therapeutic manifestation

Nevertheless, I am assuming the possibility that aesthetic practice can bear upon the political, personal and therapeutic aspects of life. This does not mean, in this context, the use of art as therapy – as in 'art therapy' – for the simple reason that the institutionalisation of art runs against the grain of the work I want to consider. Works of illness are more often made outside of medicine, sometimes in opposition to it, but always with the aim of 'saying something' about the world that illness has opened up for the afflicted persons.

Nothing here is guaranteed in terms of 'therapy', a matter that is significant but cannot be assumed prior to examining the particular. Whatever the case with particular works, the idea that art in general is made with the aim of remedy is questionable. Of course, people paint and write in the cause of expressing something about their suffering, but these are not the same thing. The link here with religion is historically contingent in that, following the decline of religious belief, art has been argued to replace it in offering hope. Quoting Nietzsche, "We possess art lest we perish from the truth", O'Toole has suggested that art offers not truth but illusion. So,

> The anxiety and terror provoked by evil, suffering, time, and death must be suppressed by a faith and confidence in life which, in the modern age, can derive only from the aesthetic realm. ... It proclaims the dignity and significance of humanity by its affirmation and celebration of existence and ultimately renders life endurable (O'Toole, 1996: 132)

This is a sweeping claim but is given a new twist in a world where medical science increasingly offers probabilities and risks, the taking of which are held to be the responsibility of the patient. It certainly holds out the promise that works of illness are important, that they give meaning even where they have no function. Sontag places this in context when she said that:

> The writer is the exemplary sufferer because he has found the deepest level of suffering and also the professional means to sublimate ... his suffering. As a man he suffers; as a writer, he transforms his suffering

> into art. The writer is the man who discovers the use of suffering in the
> economy of art – as the saints discovered the utility and necessity of
> suffering in the economy of salvation. (Sontag, 1961: 42)

In a commentary that foreshadows her discontent with the postmodern obsession with 'health' some forty years later, Sontag undoes a naïve reading of this passage by pointing out that the writer's role is historically linked to the modernist search for 'self'. What she terms 'an insatiable modern preoccupation with psychology' (1961: 42), takes the form of attempts to infuse the self with feeling, resulting in a special fascination for making works of art and the 'venture of sexual love' as 'the two most exquisite sources of suffering' (1961: 48). It is not that the writer is granted, in essence, the role of exemplary sufferer, but that we live in a world where readers seek in novels and other literature that image of their 'selves' that characterises the feelings they seek to recapture.

In a postmodern world, the different narratives and sheer plurality of voices is what distinguishes its take on suffering from that of the modernist vision. In an argument that can serve as a guide to the views put forward in this book, David Morris (1998) has pointed out that this plurality must be expressed within cultural forms – genres – if we are to learn to read it. And these forms change, so that tragedy that once bound characters to their fate is now worked through in novels that engage the reader as witness rather than detached observer. The revolt against the fate of illness is fashioned along new lines, making new claims and establishing spaces for new arguments about illness and its treatment.

Morris concludes that the challenge for a postmodern culture is 'to find genres appropriate for our era that validate, illuminate and authenticate suffering – especially the easily ignored suffering of minority groups – while seeking to alleviate and oppose it' (1998: 216-217). If old or new genres about suffering are considered remedial, then they attain this potential historically, culturally, and by that measure aesthetically. Writing, photography and painting are ways of cultivating the depiction of suffering, not in order to suppress or diminish it, but, imaginatively, through testimony and witness, to engage and express it.

This quest for new genres would seem to fit squarely with examining how 'works of illness' might also be 'works of freedom'. The question that arises then is, do stories and pictures validate, illuminate and authenticate suffering, and if so how is this achieved? This question points in two directions, one towards the social setting in which works are created and understood, and the other towards the cultural forms themselves.

In the chapters to follow I will take up each of these two lines of inquiry. Chapter 2 begins by examining the social contexts in which pictures and stories about illness are made in order to make change. This includes art made in the cause of raising public consciousness; of improving the situation of the ill; of influencing those in authority; and in establishing local support through concerted action. In Chapter 3 the argument is made that works of illness are also made to influence in a different way; not to make change in the structures or processes of society but in the way that other individuals think about the situation of the ill person. While no less social, this endeavour concerns the re-creation of the ill person's experience for another; to use a shorthand, this is the art of witness, in which the response to the ill person is less spurred by indignation (for the cause of their suffering) than by a compassionate response that seeks to acknowledge and to understand it.

Having discussed the social contexts of production and reception of works of illness, I turn in Chapter 4 to the potential for stories and pictures to have a therapeutic or revolutionary role for person making the work. The idea of redemption covers these two possibilities, raising questions about the role of such works in the lives of people who create them, often in the face of serious disease and sometimes a terminal prognosis. The question here is how works are, in a sense, life sustaining, and what bearing this possibility has on how others perceive them.

In Chapters 5 and 6 I turn to the idea of 'the cultural forms themselves', by which I mean examining the way that stories and pictures about serious illness are 'made up', are given form so that they do a particular kind of work. First, in Chapter 5 I examine the response to stories (more so pictures) that people find difficult because they deal with matters of disease, pain, decay and death. In short, this chapter takes up the issue of horror, not merely as a response to difficult pictures, but as something that necessarily precedes the fabrication of works. A key idea is that such works involve conveying, in transmuted form, horrors that have been passed through. By sketching out how stories and pictures of illness signify, this chapter sets up the requirement for how these cultural forms are deemed to be effective.

Chapter 6 puts forward an analysis of how stories and pictures about illness are 'made up', the conventions used and the ways of signifying that enable the author or artist to communicate their world. It is a 'world of illness' into which the viewer or reader is ushered, invited, drawn (even if reluctantly). It is because this communication engages the senses (because it is aesthetic, as well as political, ethical) that it makes such stories and pictures individually compelling and culturally significant.

Addressing illness experience in these terms meets the test that Osborne (1997) sets sociology, while opening up the aesthetic dimension as a way of approaching how illness is configured in the modern world. We need to be prepared to go into this in some detail if we are to emerge from the analysis with something that we can use more widely. We are searching here for nothing less than a different way of talking about illness, a way that acknowledges that the representation of suffering involves world-making, not just acts of interpretation and social judgement.

Chapter 2

Illness Activism:
making visible, finding a voice

Stories are often told and depictions shown with the intention of heightening interest in or deepening a concern for the situation of the ill, so that the aesthetic qualities of the works are a vehicle for their message, not the primary aim of the communication. Without endorsing the implication that the aesthetic is a mere vehicle of meaning, I want to explore how such works are taken up and used by fellow sufferers and by others in the cause of sharing and extending ideas about illness.

This line of thinking places the emphasis upon stories and pictures being made to influence and to encourage. They do not merely indicate something, transmute or even disarm (in the case of illness, perhaps, are therapeutic). By the same token, all artworks exist in a political world. Stories and pictures are taken up within social movements that use them to further their aims, to spread their message and to anchor images so that people can rally around central or common ideas. The question then arises, 'what is the relationship of the aesthetic and political dimensions of works of illness?'

Another way of asking this question is to enquire into the practices by which the aesthetic and the political are fashioned and recognised as aspects of works, and the means by which one might overshadow the other? Under what circumstances – and with what aim – might a picture or account be taken as an icon or tract rather than an artwork, and vice-versa. These are important questions, given that many artists and authors have been explicit about the fact that they wrote, painted or photographed to improve things for people suffering with serious illness. However, these questions are also important because social movements make use of stories and pictures in order to better the situation of the ill. As a result, these works attain a new and widened sphere of significance. The intentions of individual authors and artists are surpassed, by which I mean not overridden, but realised through acclaim, protest and dialogue. We need to inquire into how such artworks change the world and how they are changed as a result, as well as remembering that they are fashioned in an existing political climate and social order.

To illustrate that an appreciation of the artist's aim – or the artwork's expressive thrust – is not inevitable, I want to examine two stories about attempts to publicise illness told by the British photographer Jo Spence. In an interview with David Hevey (1992: 125-6) she described what she called 'the peak of my experience as a cancer patient'. At the end of a conference of self-help groups where she showed her '*Picture of Health*' exhibition, she was helped to take it down by two women who asked her 'why she was so angry'. When she answered that there was a lot to be angry about, the women countered with the reply, 'But they're doing the best they can', where 'they' referred to members of the medical profession. The women said that they could not deal with things ideologically but only in terms of practicalities that would facilitate adapting to the situation in which they found themselves. Not being able to 'deal with things ideologically' meant that they could not discern Spence's question, 'How is our illness represented and how does that help to position us through our basic ignorance?' The idea that illness is already represented (i.e. it already positions, is already ideological) is facilitated by the exhibition of images that are born of the imagination. On this occasion, the mundane political world of the women patients was resistant to the ideological challenge offered by Spence, while her aesthetic offering was marginalized completely.

In case this story implies that the aesthetic dimension of Spence's photographs was entirely overlooked, she told of the fate of this exhibition in another context. Recalling its reception at a gallery opening, she spoke of the 'amazing silence' with which it was met, 'except for someone coming up and saying, "I like the green card it's on". This is a revealing comment not just for its banality, but also for the way it shows how aesthetic features (even if only supporting ones) can be foregrounded by separating them from signs belonging to the mundane world. Comments about the artistic qualities of works on show are to be expected at a gallery exhibition, but it is again the absence of recognition of the ideological content that is noteworthy here. In this case it is the aesthetic dimension – legitimated by context – which is used to marginalize the political, and ultimately *aestheticize* the works on show. As in the previous context, the result was that the status quo regarding illness remained resistant to Spence's ideological challenge.

In both situations it is Spence's ideological imagination that is subjugated by the separation of the political and the aesthetic. This might be taken as a lesson in the plasticity of interpretation, underlining the point that what is 'made' of a work depends upon context, and upon the interests of those who view and/or read it (Becker, 1988). Certainly Spence was of the view that the audience for her work was important, and this was underlined by the response of women with breast cancer to whom she showed her photographs. About this she said:

> When the work goes to places where people have cancer, there's no taboo at all, they just fall about you with open arms and say, "How marvellous to be able to talk about it. That we could talk about having a breast removed or being badly damaged by surgery or our hair dropping out or whatever". So, it's the difference between audiences: if you put it into one context, it's bad art, you put it into another context, it's brilliant information. (Spence, in Hevey, 1992: 123).

The interpretation of photographs such as these by women with breast cancer is not just context dependent, as Spence seems to suggest here, but also context making. These works make a difference to viewers (who 'fall about you with open arms') because they have both aesthetic and political potential. Such photographs encourage dialogue and enable relationships to be established in which common concerns can be articulated and related to the works on show. This, in turn, involves articulating a renewed significance in the light of the dialogue they have fostered. The photographs come to matter – to matter more – and this endows them with a meaning tied to their potential to enable people to talk about difficult experiences. So it is not merely how works are interpreted that is important here, but how they come to be made different in the course of being taken up by others. In discussing this, we need to move to a position that sees artworks as being part of an emerging culture of illness, not just being affected by such a culture or in turn merely influencing it. And to see how works play that part we have to link discussion of the social and political with the form of signification within them. To call this 'interpretation' falls short of the mark, because it involves changes in the way that viewers and readers relate *to each other* through engaging the work. It also concerns the ways that people then relate *to the work* by virtue of their changed relationship to each other. Part of this latter relationship might well involve how ill people identify themselves and address the world of the healthy. Conceived politically, stories and pictures about illness are about addressing boundaries that imply not merely difference but inequality, and sometimes stigma as well.

This elaboration of meaning not only happens in situations where the artist/writer and the sufferer are the same person, but also in situations where the artist/writer is a third party. This is a useful distinction to make at this point because we need to examine the conditions under which people (audiences) respond 'at a distance' so to speak. This is not only in terms of limits in shared background experience (not everyone who looks at Spence's pictures is a woman, or has breast cancer) but also in terms of the special conditions applying where the artist and the sufferer are the same person. Both of the former separations imply a distance that is to be overcome, which distance raises questions that will help illuminate the special circumstance of the autobiography or the self-portrait. It is to the question of distance that we turn in the next section.

Indignation, Pity and the Aesthetic

The idea of distance immediately raises questions of disinterestedness in a world where resistance to fate is a recognised and valued reaction. How can one be disinterested at the news that someone close to you has been diagnosed with a serious disease such as AIDS/HIV or cancer? To be ill with serious disease no longer means suffering alone or in silence, now that there has emerged so many groups that provide support for sufferers and have established a basis for political action. This is particularly so where disease has been coupled with minority group status, for example in the case of AIDS and the gay community or else breast cancer and women. We are perhaps less surprised today by a response of anger to disease than by an attitude of complacency or resignation. This is in no small part the result of the activism of the gay community in the 1980s in response to the social response (or lack of it) to AIDS and the organisation of women in the 1990s and beyond to the prevalence of breast cancer. In both of these cases, people with AIDS and women with breast cancer expressed their anger while organising politically to change public attitudes and government policy (Batt 1994; Butler and Rosenblum 1991; Crimp, 1992; Crimp and Rolston, 1990; Patten, 1998; Lorde 1980; Potts 2000).

Against this background, it is questionable whether adopting an aesthetic attitude to works of illness has merit, either in terms of the immediate benefits to the ill person or the longer-term removal of the disease from the population. Taking this a step further, one can question, on the one hand, the conditions of production of the work and, on the other, the kind of social relationship such works might produce. What is the point of art in a war against AIDS – where the aim is to mobilise resources to find a cure? Douglas Crimp (1992: 132) has asked the question, 'what is the stake of the artist in such a project?' making the claim that some artists 'traffic in the aura' attaching to art and art photography. This points up the idea that taking an aesthetic attitude toward art in the context of illness both draws away from the situation of ill people concerned, while at the same time establishing a relationship of specular distance between the observer and the work itself. For example, the relationship of the viewer to the person portrayed (e.g. a person with AIDS) is thereby limited by the way that the work was produced through a process of appropriation, where the complexity of living with AIDS is subordinated to the medium of representation.

Along similar lines, it has been said about the politics of representation that, 'the subjective aspect of liberal aesthetics is compassion rather than collective struggle. Pity, mediated by an appreciation of "great art", supplants political understanding' (Sekula, 1978: 875). The problem with this analysis is that it conflates pity with compassion, where these terms refer to different relationships between observers and observed, between the afflicted and the non-afflicted. Historically, pity as an institutionalised response (as charity) accorded particular groups a marginal place in society *as it excluded them*, be they 'cripple', 'mad' or 'leper'. These terms traditionally identified and located these individuals as being at a distance from the able-bodied spectator. What pity and collective struggle have in common – and which distinguishes them from compassion – is that both are established on a community interest with the suffering and the oppressed (Arendt, 1973). While both compassion and pity have their limitations with respect to alleviating distress, no comprehensive understanding of suffering can be made without examination of these different responses to its manifestation and its portrayal.

Before taking up this issue in more detail, we should note what has also been said about art in this context – 'the aesthetic values of the traditional art world are of little consequence to AIDS activists' (Crimp and Rolston, 1990: 16). This quote resonates with the view that any work that detracts from the life-context of the person depicted must be wanting. What has been called the denial of the particular has been noted in writers valuing the aesthetic, who it has been said, 'valorize abstract concepts and formal features' in their attempt to universalize modes of perception (Bohls, 1993). The question remains as to whether all writing about aesthetics in the context of illness falls into this trap. Do all attempts at art in the context of activism fall so short of their aim (to depict truthfully, to communicate a semblance) as to be a handicap? On the other hand, is a work that achieves Deleuze and Guattari's criterion for art (something that can 'stand up on their own', 1994: 164) enhanced if seen as iconic of the struggles of a social movement? And is a politically productive work, one that makes a social difference, more or less likely to have its aesthetic qualities sidelined as a result?

This last point leads us to ask – from which position does a political criticism of the aesthetic spring? Is it from a mode of action that is at odds with contemplation or distance in its need to organise and move towards change in the mundane world? This mode does not dispense with depiction, but in using it differently, engages with the aesthetic so as to subordinate it. To address this issue, I want briefly to examine the relationship of feelings of indignation to social organisation and modes of representation, making use of the work of Luc Boltanski (1999).

Boltanski drew upon Hannah Arendt's (1973) analysis in which she argued that pity is an orientation to the needy in which they are understood *in their generality* to be different from others. The response to pity is solidarity, and the historical response to disadvantage has been organised relief, reaching out from a distance, so creating lasting institutions that mediate between them. From the point of view of those who occupy positions of advantage – in relation to good health or otherwise – whether pity will translate into action depends upon their perception of the legitimacy of need in those afflicted. To the extent that people are seen as having brought about their own suffering, or are capable of overcoming it by themselves, then they are less likely to be seen as deserving help. In this regard, different diseases, and those afflicted by them, evoke different responses. Gay men or prostitutes with AIDS, for example, have been perceived as being responsible for their illnesses. While they might, among certain people, evoke pity – as directed toward an inferior – they might not evoke compassion, or indignation that translates into remedial and ultimately political action.

For the moment it is important to note that, in a world of politics, the aggregation and mass deployment of compassionate acts presents modern society with a problem. When people act *en masse* as in protest against the establishment, when they invade the spaces of those who would administer their just rewards and beneficence, then they eradicate, in their very presence, the distance that pity demands for its operation. Pity is a discriminating modality, and the refusal of the dispossessed to be outsiders means that they are transformed into '*les enragés*' (Arendt, 1973: 111; Boltanski, 1999: 13.). Whether this is desirable is itself a political judgment of the moment, but its manifestation tests the stability of the political structures that mediate relationships through which the dispossessed are allowed to articulate their need.

While it is not correct to say that pity can be reduced to the political, the distance that pity takes with respect to the disadvantaged as a group or class (its 'coldness') distinguishes it from compassion that accompanies the relief of suffering at hand. This can be understood when we examine what happens when those who organise do so, if not in the name of pity, then in order to overcome it under the guidance of principle and justice. Boltanski argues that a 'politics of pity' must fulfil a double requirement. It aspires to a generality in which the human condition (the dignity of the suffering) is addressed, and yet it must keep hold of individual cases that might evoke compassion. This is relevant to any discussion of art in the political context because it highlights how these two ways of being sensitised can never quite be separated from one another. Or rather, it highlights how a 'politics of pity' depends upon the retention of some spectacle of individual suffering in order that the flame of compassion is not dimmed entirely. So it is that we speak of the need to raise money, administer relief efficiently and disburse funds or goods fairly, *and yet* must retain 'compassion' for the afflicted as we do it. If this were not the case then charitable action becomes cold indeed, so that the surpassing of pity as sentiment yet requires the space, and the opportunity, for at least a semblance of compassionate response.

Clearly, the distance between actor and sufferer that is created by a politics of pity should not be confused with the ascetic distance of the aesthetic attitude. Aesthetics, like compassion and pity, can be taken as another topic whose application is not entirely separable from these other two, as we shall see in the following chapter. This is important in our discussion of the role of art in illness activism where the analysis of the scope and sphere of representation requires that we be sensitive to the mutual overlap of these three topics. However, to do this we need recourse to examples from the world of illness experience, activism and representation, examples that we shall take below. At this point, where we are concerned with protest arising from illness, it is to indignation that we look in search of clues as to the role of artworks in establishing, refining or challenging pity. What, if anything, is depicted by ill people who would not be pitied or denied their rights, and in the cause of promoting which kinds of sentiments?

Illness, Activism and Representation

When one thinks of the banners and the paintings, the poems and the plays, collective actions and associated artefacts, not to mention the wealth of photographs and videos that have been the stuff of protest, then it is clear that an appreciation of the 'aesthetics of illness' needs to be set in some political and historical context. A vital part of this is the recognition that protest emerged from existing inequalities and the ways these were recruited to the public response to disease. With respect to AIDS/HIV, male homosexual and lesbian communities were involved in attempts to counter stigma that they saw as emanating from the mass media, to confront medicine in its designation of risk-categories and to challenge directly the middle-class (American) establishment on its own ground (Gamson, 1989; Griffin, 2000). It is not surprising that the protest group ACT UP (AIDS Coalition to Unleash Power) used direct action in the form of theatre, much of it testing the bounds of 'good taste'. Making use of strategies of political protest that had been employed by feminists amongst others, ACT UP created what Patten calls 'a theatre of our bodies in the public sphere' (1998: 390). In one protest, women put on hospital gowns, and dragged mattresses through the streets of Chicago to highlight the plight of women with AIDS waiting for treatment in the local hospital. The purpose of events like this was to make a visual homology of the activists' identification and solidarity with the women concerned. The symbolic meaning of the mattresses lay in the number of unfilled beds in the hospital while the protestors' visibility attested not only to the situation of people with AIDS but also the readiness of this wider group to speak out on their behalf. Performance of this kind both depicts and claims at the same time, so that it deploys some of the ways in which art signifies (through depiction, through metaphor) but within the context of a particular political message. Its other aim was to challenge the 'immunity' from AIDS that the message of the mass media had created for its readership, in an attempt to implicate the mainstream American culture, if not into its way of life, then into its way of death (Goldstein, 1991).

Drawing upon the ideas of the European photographer John Heartfield (Roberts, 1998), AIDS activists often used text alongside images, or imaged text, to make their messages more direct and linked to the everyday life of the 'immune' whom they would implicate in their situation. During the inter-war years Heartfield had juxtaposed everyday images (e.g. of goods in shops, the poor) with political slogans to highlight the plight of working people in German society. The use of text in art and the use of images alongside text are mutually supporting, and for activists with a commitment to change it was the inclusion of text that was of major importance. This derived from a view of art as being grounded in ideological struggles rather than it being an objectification of personal vision. From this perspective art is harnessed to a political agenda so that the aesthetic – the shocking, the bad taste – becomes the thrust in an argument aimed at social change. And particularly important in this context, it is the borrowing of images from mainstream society and then subverting them that does the work of drawing in observers and provoking a response.

In its subversion of mainstream material culture ACT UP used elements of depiction that extended to what mainstream culture might call 'bad taste', or what gallery curators would consider less than art. Visual symbols were created through appropriation, such as the image "SILENCE = DEATH" written in bold white-on-black letters beneath a pink triangle. This image came to signify AIDS activism to a wide group of people, its appropriation a sign of the power of graphics to promote solidarity. The pink triangle – now upright rather than inverted – had been a symbol for homosexuals used by the Nazis. This image was reproduced on a number of items. In one example beneath the main text were the words: 'Why is Reagan silent about AIDS? What is really going on at the Center for Disease Control, the Federal Drug Administration, and the Vatican? Gays and lesbian are not expendable…Use your power…Vote…Boycott…Defend yourselves…Turn anger, fear, grief into action.' (Crimp and Rolston, 1990: 29).

Other images were more transgressive in their placing of gay interests at the centre of the AIDS campaign. In her account of her involvement in the ACT UP movement, Mary Patten (1998) describes how, 'We sketched a woman going down on another woman, sandwiched between the words "Power Breakfast" printed in large italicised bold gothic type, a la Barbara Kruger'. (1998: 396) What is interesting about this image (says Patten) is that while it provoked a negative reaction among some women (and men) who saw it as degrading to women, others saw it sufficiently positively for it to become ACT UP's best selling T-shirt in years to come. This set the scene for the commodification of images and designs that arguably have marked the maturation of social movements relating to social resistance. Having borrowed images and aspects of commodity culture (the T-shirt) to promote their message, the ACT UP movement put in place (in the marketplace) designs whose aesthetic appeal aligned with the messages of social justice being put forward. This alignment can be seen as a form of public, social positioning, in which by wearing a T-shirt one announces one's support for the cause.

In this way, over time, even ordinary (and less transgressive items) such as ribbons and buttons could be bought by anyone who would identify with a cause at a distance. This is a movement of thinking, from art to "queer style", where the purchase of a red or pink ribbon eventually becomes an ornamental marker of individual identity and lifestyle choice as an AIDS or breast cancer aware person (Moore, 2008). This mainstreaming is not restricted to the selling of ornaments. Where charities used AIDS associated artworks either in the cause of raising awareness or in fundraising there was a tendency to abstract the disease way from its socio-political context through framing AIDS as a tragic disease of individuals (Engberg, 1991). This points up the ambiguous and unstable status of works that can be re-framed in order to move them further away from their political origin. In the modern world this does not mean having to choose between making works into either 'art' (in a gallery) or into artefacts for sale in a shop. The world that Benjamin (1970) anticipated enables such images to be reproduced on the T-shirt or the poster, but with consequences for dispersing if not diluting political power, as compared with the diminishing of aura. The commodification of images has meant, if anything, the aestheticization of politics, along with the politicization of art (Foster, 1985). In this way, aesthetics enters – or re-enters – illness though another door to that which one might expect with respect to activist art.

Politically inspired artworks aim to make visible an alternative or hidden aspect of the social system or of social groups. This aim can be contrasted with the idea that art should represent the unknowable, the impossible to reveal (the sublime). The hidden aspects in the case of AIDS were the lesbian, gay and queer identities, the battle for which was seen by some activists as identical with the war on AIDS (Patten, 1998). However, it is wrong to suggest a dichotomy between the politically real and the aesthetically sublime, if only because representations of illness do (as Adorno (1984) claimed for art) achieve their meaning (their control) by virtue of ideas in the sphere of the mundane. It is with reference to the world of things and ideas that art owes its powers. In the introduction to their photo project, *Positive Lives: Responses to HIV*, Mayes and Stein (1993) made a case for photography being able to present an emotional immediacy that transcends the reality of the moment. This is against the background of their argument that AIDS (as with any illness) defies picturing, but that the social and political context that developed around it can be shown. Mayes and Stein's case that AIDS is special is built upon the observation that, as a medical condition, it received (at that time) more treatment in print than in direct services to those afflicted. While this is no longer true, the special conditions attaching to AIDS do not make it a disease on its own, as we shall see below. In one sense, Mayes and Stein's claim draws on the kinds of arguments that have been made for photography in general over the years, not least in this regard by John Berger (see Berger and Mohr, 1989). And yet their argument opens up the wider implication that serious illness of any kind has differential effects upon people depending upon the social situation in which they live. As already mentioned, the 'otherness' of people afflicted with disease will affect the readiness of people to respond to them – to feel pity for them – so that indignation does not spring ready made from the mere viewing of a picture of despair. The group identity of the person pictured, their relationship to mainstream society, perceived culpability for their present situation and their ability to help themselves are matters that underlie the propensity for the viewer to feel indignation and to act to relieve suffering (Radley and Kennedy, 1997).

Straddling the supposed divide between reality and representation is the documentary, of which several were made at the time when there was a struggle to bring AIDS to mainstream attention. One reason for the use of video in conjunction with protest is that it provided visual records of events that, for better or worse, were treated as unvarnished reality (Holden, 2000). In her review of alternative media coverage of AIDS, Juhasz (1995) made the comparison between documentary and science. Drawing upon the work of Nichols she argues that documentaries made about AIDS (rather than made by people with AIDS) share with science a pleasure in control through knowledge. To quote Nichols:

> Documentary realism aligns itself with an *epistephilia*, so to speak, a pleasure in knowing, that marks out a distinctive form of social engagement. The engagement stems from the rhetorical force of an argument about the very world we inhabit. We are moved to confront a topic, issue, situation, or event that bears the mark of the historically real. In igniting our interest, a documentary has a less incendiary effect on our erotic fantasies and sense of sexual identity but a stronger effect on our social imagination and sense of cultural identity. (Nichols, 1991: 178)

Nichols is arguing that documentary, as well as art, involves pleasure, but pleasure of a different sort. Where art engages us in the pleasures of looking (erotics), documentary offers us the pleasures of knowing (epistephilia). And where art follows this by raising questions about the accomplishment of semblance, documentary first answers questions of veracity and legitimacy in order to produce the pleasures of knowing. This viewpoint is clearly different to that created by the artist, who renders the world in an imaginary way, or perhaps more accurately, renders imaginary worlds that viewers might inhabit. The maker of a documentary is taken (by the viewer) to operate from inside the historically real world, making a representation of the same world that s/he (and we) can be said to occupy. The issue in judging documentary film is therefore not the quality of the imaginary world so created (how good an artwork is it?) but how has the filmmaker acquitted herself or himself in relation to the film produced? This concerns issues to do with the standpoint, argument and politics of the director – in short it concerns the *ethics* of filmmaking.

This distinction between the 'ethics of documentary' and the 'erotics of art' invites us to ask further questions about the way that illness is represented, not least by activists in relation to particular diseases. However, this inevitably begs the question as to whether video and still photography can be separated neatly into art and documentary. For our purposes in this book, the distinction between erotics and ethics leads to questions about the way that these matters have deliberately or accidentally been introduced in works that represent illness experience. While these points will be taken up later on, it is useful to note that illness narratives made as text or as video are primarily documents, and so concern ethics. While they are able to tell a story within the story, or otherwise evoke worlds that might have been, they too partake of the sublime, if not the erotic. For example, the film made by Judith Helfand, titled "A Healthy Baby Girl," is a documentary in which Helfand is the narrator, central character and author. Helfand suffered from vaginal cancer as a result of her mother having taken the drug diethylstilbestrol (DES), prescribed to prevent miscarriage during the 1940s to the 1970s. Susan Bell's analysis of this film emphasises:

> ... the extent to which this visual narrative so skilfully draws together a complex relationship between Judith and her mother and father infused with the promise of DES and trauma of DES cancer along with the public issues of medicine's golden age and pharmaceutical manufacturers. (Bell, 2004)

This suggests an interweaving of public issues, of ethical issues to do with prescription, treatment and mothering. However, the film also uses stylistic devices – including music – to evoke feelings to do with the fact that Judith's mother was the unwitting agent of her daughter's illness and its consequences

> The repetition of the words "they had taken something from me" and "they had given something back to her" as the first words in the film underscore their importance and encourage us to fill in the "they" and the "something" (and perhaps the "I" and "her") ... That she follows this with a scene of herself, clothed, sitting in front of a fireplace and gesturing, how, with the word "and that's where I guess our experiences kind of divide" looking straight at viewers, using her hands for emphasis, "thickens" for me the meaning she is communicating of the complicated relationship she has (and had) with her mother, of their gains and losses, of her aloneness and connection with her mother. This interpretation gains strength with the sound, now, of a one-fingered lullaby – evoking lullabies played and hummed by Judith's mother, heard and felt by Judith. The music, though, takes Judith's and her mother's experiences beyond their individual lives and connects them to Jewish tradition and family life. ... In addition, the lullaby connects Judith and her mother to audiences' experiences of humming, singing, playing lullabies; and to hearing and feeling lullabies being sung. (Bell, 2004).

In this quote Bell directs attention to something that is communicated about mother-daughter relationships that is not locatable 'in' the film, in the sense that it is not circumscribed in talk or by reference to place. The film is, if anything, expressive of that relationship, so painfully turned by the insertion of the drug into Judith's mother's pregnancy. There are moments, in this documentary, where the satisfaction of watching it comes not from knowing about, but in being 'witness to'. Judith Helfand's film is autobiographical, so that one might argue that it is different in important respects from mainstream documentary made about ill people, rather than by them. This point is a reminder that to document is different to (but not exclusive from) rendering in an imaginary way.

To illustrate this, consider a more recent case of activism regarding a disease that strikes (though not exclusively) women – breast cancer. In a recent article, Brown, et al. (2004) point to the ways that the environmental breast cancer movement has constructed what they term 'a politicised collective illness identity' through transforming individual illness experience, critiquing medicine's treatment of women patients, and turning attention away from women's bodies as sites of risk to the environment in which they live. Examples of locations in which this transformation take place include the internet, where women with breast cancer share experiences and also try to help other women prevent themselves from falling ill (Pitts 2004; Sharf

1997); public spaces where women organise races, walks and touring events that '…produce and transform the emotions that create solidarity and strengthen participation' in collective action (Klawiter, 2000: 69); science education projects 'initiated and designed by activists working with experts (Braun 2003); and the circulation among women's groups of films that address issues to do with mastectomy, family and sexual relationships (Butler and Rosenblum 1993; Cartwright 1998; Onwura 1991).

Making breast cancer public involves making breast cancer visible, something designed to breach the cultural cloak that has lain over both cancer in general and breast cancer in particular. The making visible of this disease, its consequences and its context, has been achieved by what Klawiter (2000), following Swidler (1995) has called 'ritual practices' that lead to a political vision anchored in a set of interpretations of women's bodies.

The use of visual images showing women's bodies bearing the scars of mastectomy has been a rallying point in different contexts. Klawiter describes how, in one demonstration in San Francisco, women held high exhibits of photographs of women's nude torsos, including 'startling images of disfigured women with double mastectomies' (2000: 85). In another walk in support of breast cancer action one woman ('an exhibitionist') wears a dress with one half pulled down at the front to reveal the evidence of her breast cancer history. Another woman – seeing this – removes her shirt to show the asymmetry of her chest. Klawiter interprets this as 'a practice of participation that works on and through bodies' (2000: 88). This practice – a movement from 'below' rather than from the ideology of institutions – involves social relations, discourses and regulatory actions, which together constitute a change in what Klawiter (2004) calls the *disease regime* of breast cancer. Although disease regimes are relatively structured and stable, they are subject to a wide variety of cross-cutting pressures (Klawiter, 2004: 850). As she argues, some social movements (and breast cancer is one) 'achieve their greatest impact in the cultural arena, through changing popular images, ideas, emotions and identities' (Klawiter, 2004: 851). As part of this, visual images are key in rendering visible and collective the shared experience of being a woman with breast cancer.

Some of these images are more durable than others. An early example of a lasting image is poet Deena Metzger's 'The Warrior' (1977), (photograph by Hella Hammid, also known as "Tree Poster," designed by Sheila Levrant de Bretteville), which has been reproduced in more than twenty publications, including the feminist health 'bible' *Our Bodies, Ourselves*, as well as in postcards, and posters, and the world wide web (http://www.deena metzger.com/poster/poster.html) (see Sharf 1997). In this black and white photograph, Metzger is standing outside, shot from below so that viewers look up at her nude torso. Her face is in profile, looking up, smiling, towards the sky. Her arms are outstretched against the sky behind and above her, openly showing her bare chest. Her right breast is missing. The photo is cropped at hip level. A tattoo of a tree branch covers her scar, running from her armpit almost to the centre of her chest. This tattoo includes grape leaves on a vine, the Book of Life, and a bird (Van Schaick 1998). Metzer's image invites the world to look and to see a one-breasted woman, and other one-breasted women to see 'The Warrior.'

A more recent example is the use of the model Matuschka's self-portrait, 'Beauty Out of Damage,' showing her mastectomy scar, on the cover of the *New York Times Magazine* (August 15, 1993). The author of the piece – Susan Ferraro – had seen some of Matuschka's images at a rally organised to "fight against breast cancer". This picture struck a powerful chord with readers at the time, even though it was controversial. Matuschka (1993) explains on her web site how she had been working on images like this since she learned of her diagnosis, and emphasises how, in trying to get it published, it was "Middle America" she wanted to reach. But even alongside this, she sought to make "beautiful pictures" from her marked body, with the result that when she succeeded, she thought: "now I can make art out of *anything* (emphasis in the original). Even as Matuschka 'reclaim[ed] the scar as an object of aesthetic and political significance and, more profoundly, as an object of fascination, if not beauty' (Cartwright, 1998: 128), her white, youthful and sophisticated appearance actually inhibited her acceptance by many women. This is because visual images of women with mastectomies draw upon different representations of race, age and social class. What made her image a public icon of breast cancer was her role as conventional model, art photographer and activist-by–default. We can see here that judgements about what is art and what makes good activist photos are not entirely separable if only for the reason that these judgements often rely upon each other.

An Example of 'activist art' – the 'Obsessed with Breasts' Campaign

In 2000 the *Breast Cancer Fund of America* created a poster campaign based in San Francisco aimed at raising consciousness both of the disease and of their own website. The posters (see Figure 1 for an example) showed pictures of scantily clad young women (models), in stereotyped poses, revealing mastectomy scars, with the accompanying text, "It's no secret" and "Obsessed with breasts". The colour photographs were made by 'grafting' on pictures of real mastectomy scars on to the bodies of the models. Created by an advertising agency, the posters mimicked the style of well-known advertisers of lingerie and perfume, so that the glamour borrows from women's magazines while the poses (with the chest revealed) echo the pages of a men's soft-porn publication.

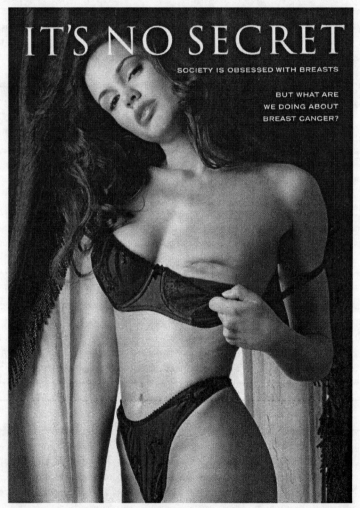

Figure 1. *'It's No Secret'. Image from the Breast Cancer Fund's Obsessed with Breasts advertising campaign, 2000, used with permission. www.breastcancerfund.org*

The key goals of the campaign were:

> To increase awareness and involve the public in breast cancer issues.
> To replace fear of the disease with the desire to act.
> To educate and provide ways for people to act.
> To prompt and answer questions from children and young adults about the disease.

The plan was to show the 'advertisements' in approximately 30 bus shelters, for six weeks beginning mid-January 2000. However, the posters were refused by the San Francisco bus shelter authorities, which feared shocking the public. As a result Santa Clara officials took them down after three complaints had been made. This provoked public outrage, and considerable press coverage. The Breast Cancer Fund reported on their website that 'a poll in the Contra Costa Times (of the east Bay) showed 79% in favor of keeping the posters up', and 19 of the original 23 ads that were posted in the East Bay shelters remained up for their allotted time.

Figure 1 shows one of the 'advertisements', which parodies the cover of a well-known women's magazine. The picture shows a model posing in her underwear, exposing a mastectomy scar on her chest. The model's pose mimics those adopted by models on the front covers of women's magazines, and is accompanied by text that echoes that format. The title is "IT'S NO SECRET", and below this announces SOCIETY IS OBSESSED WITH BREASTS, and BUT WHAT ARE WE DOING ABOUT BREAST CANCER? The 'Obsessed with Breasts' campaign exploited the experience of organisations such as ACT UP to 'get the public's attention' by their shocking representation of womanhood. They did this by juxtaposing, in the same picture, images designed to elicit desire with those designed to elicit abhorrence. This was done with the expectation that by de-mystifying breast cancer it would hold less threat for members of the public. This approach rests upon the assumption that by making visible the scars of treatment, the disease becomes something that can be dealt with. Hence, the potential for the posters to provoke indignation was as important as the potential to inform or to convey ideas of empowerment.

These depictions engage the viewer through the tropes normally associated with breasts as objects of sexual desire. While the organisation reported support for the campaign in the order of about 7 to 1, inspection of the website reveals a variety of objections to the pictures (Breast Cancer Fund, 2000). These included commentators who saw the pictures as 'too strong, graphic and sexual to be displayed where the public [and especially children] can see them', and those who took issue with the frightening images depicted; 'these ads are horrible!! Am I supposed to be eager to seek treatment of possible breast cancer knowing I might look like that? How about ads showing survivors in a positive way? Cancer is scary enough!' It is not made clear as to whether the commentators are men or women, but the sense from reading them is that it was women who wrote in.

This matters because the discordance of the pictures is likely to be different for men and women, certainly those who are heterosexual. Women see a discrepancy in the ugliness of the scars and the beauty of the young models, with whom they can identify to a greater or lesser degree, depending on age and their own or close others' health history regarding breast cancer. For example:

> I think the posters you are planning on using are disgusting. I am a cancer survivor and my chest does not look like that. I don't want my friends or loved ones to see the posters because then every time they look at me they will see the gross chest pictures you are using. Most women in the age group you are using have re-constructive surgery done, so it is unrealistic to show those pictures. I highly resent it. (The Breast Cancer Fund, 2000).

This quote shows that images displayed in public appear for a variety of audiences, and that even those individuals directly implicated may not read the depictions in the way intended. Women vary by race, class and age, as well as by medical history, so that the view that there is a common experience that might be captured by art (activist or otherwise) is almost certainly a mistake (Cartwright, 1998).

In the case of the *Breast Cancer Fund* images this point is especially true where the audience for the posters was made up of men, especially heterosexual men. They experience a different discordance, stemming from being lured into an erotically based looking that finds an abhorrent object (the scar) that 'looks back', and in so doing undoes the scopophilia in which they are engaged. This is compounded by the elicitation of a compassionate response sought by the text, producing a kind of flicker effect in modality of looking, so that the gaze that searches for the missing breast only serves to undo itself further.

This also indicates that what pictures mean will be mediated by the degree to which viewers adhere to socially sanctioned schemes of public and private representation, something that has been fashioned by the penetration of photographic technology and practice into culture. Photographic depictions are claimed (or claim for themselves) to be a 'kind of' picture, and their acceptability, their legitimacy is judged in that light. This legitimacy is grounded in part upon what is depicted, in part upon how it was produced, and in part upon where and to whom it is shown. The 'Obsessed with Breasts' posters work (or fail, depending on one's standpoint) because they deliberately transgress everyday assumptions about the 'kind of' pictures that should serve as advertisements in public places. By identifying the posters as 'ads.' the commentators show this to be true. This is consistent with the everyday belief that illness is not a suitable subject for photography, if it is assumed that what is ugly is not deemed photographable. If photographs – or rather, the photographable – has become the criterion by which we judge what is desirable to show about *ourselves*, then by this yardstick illness is a state that disqualifies us from wishing such images to survive.

Depictions such as the '*Obsessed with Breasts*' posters are understood in relation to a set of social conventions that are, in turn, shaped in the course of picturing (Goffman, 1976). This is an important point to make lest we fall into the trap of believing that because images are subject to convention they are necessarily determined. The poster campaign of the *Breast Cancer Fund* did not merely, through shock tactics, direct people to their web site, but provided a pictorial space in which ways of seeing illness might be re-ordered. The contradiction of tropes and the juxtaposition of genres created the space for a web dialogue that, while it was about these images, was also about the place (the rights) of the sick in society. This means that how we learn to see in one genre can itself affect how we see in others, so that what begins as art might be taken over into the politics of health and vice-versa (Dykstra, 1995).

Art and Illness: the space of representation

One of the important ways in which activists have countered mainstream views of illness – or addressed the silence regarding disease – is by the occupation of space in order to transform it. This might occur through protest in which people's bodies are deployed in ways that re-inscribe those spaces, including the disruption of ongoing mainstream activities. It also occurs where people use artefacts to 'occupy' a place such as a bus shelter, or else use items like clothing that are mobile and pass through spaces where they can be seen. Finally, spaces are marked through being transformed by activities so that they become sites for imagining different possibilities. The last is perhaps best exemplified by the notion of theatre – either institutional or *ad hoc* – in which a performance made by actors tells some story – projects some vision – of the fate of people afflicted with disease.

Artworks have a special role in facilitating the transformation of space for a number of reasons, not least that they promote visibility. Visual images are important for their potential to establish significant practices surrounding a disease like AIDS or breast cancer, or to make some practices endure more than others. This issue is raised in the context of the claim that the establishment of new social practices requires 'the visible, public enactment of new patterns so that "everyone can see" that everyone else has seen that things have changed' (Swidler, 2001: 87). In the case of the AIDS and breast cancer movements this mutual seeing has also involved a mutual showing. The role of visual images in this is important as a way in which activists and others can *recognise* the issues on which the movement is grounded and use these images to formulate and share collective aims. Susan Sontag makes this point in relation to photographs, which she says, 'lay down routes of reference and serve as totems of causes: sentiment is more likely to crystallise around a photograph than around a verbal slogan' (Sontag 2003: 76). The sentiment in this case is indignation, and it serves to consolidate the group in the service of accusatory action aimed at social change. While it is a mistake to assume that all pressure groups are the same, the moral conditions attaching to illness mean that 'the collective interpretation of illness is made in terms which, in the strict sense of the wording, *challenge society or the social order*' (Herzlich, 1995: 160, emphasis in the original). We have seen that, with respect to space, this challenge is made both in terms of visibility and in terms of ideology, where the latter involves the articulation of arguments concerning the social and political conditions attaching to disease, its diagnosis and treatment. These two features are not easily distinguishable in acts of protest in a world dominated by issues of rights and justice.

Drawing directly upon Benhabib's (1990) analysis of Hannah Arendt's writings, we can determine these two uses of space as being *agonistic* and *discursive* respectively, where both refer to the public realm. Discursive space is that where 'freedom can appear', where people together share ideas and values through speech so as to counter oppression and pain. Benhabib glosses this statement in an important way for this analysis, by saying that it is not a topographical space – one defined in terms of places or crowds – but a space defined in terms of 'action in concert' (1990: 194). By comparison, the space of appearances relates to 'making visible', where moral and political signs are revealed, displayed and shared with others. It is also a space where signs compete to be seen, to invite and challenge the viewer. If as, Benhabib says, this space was important to the Romans and the Greeks as a 'guarantee against the futility of individual life', and 'promoting a relative permanence if not immortality for mortals', then its existence is no less relevant in the modern world for individuals feeling isolated when living with serious disease. Every public space has something of the agonistic and the discursive: they are not exclusive properties of action. The emancipation of the sick – which is, at one level, what AIDS and breast cancer activism strive for – is no different in making use of both types of space. Posters and photographs with text have both the power *to shock* (to make visible) and *to narrate* (to engage discursively through sign manipulation). Neither of these is reducible one to the other.

In the modern world, however, the discursive is dominant because the struggle to make something public is always the struggle for justice, the move to action out of pity. Social movements articulate a world of rights rather than appearances, even though the former makes use of the latter to make its claims. It was the deployment of images as weapons in the fight for rights of people with AIDS (as legitimated by Crimp and Rolston (1990) that unnerved some critics who wanted a more 'aesthetic' use of portrayals and depictions (see Griffin, 2000 for a discussion).

The establishment of discursive space is essentially – through its use of speech and persuasion – the creation of a public space. It brings into view matters that were previously private and contained within boundaries of family or group. For Arendt, violence (and prejudice) can appear in public or in private but its language is essentially private because it is the language of pain (Benhabib, 1990: 194; Scarry, 1985). (The violence of the afflicted person who strikes out against his or her tormentor is on a similar plane.) Pain is the stuff of illness, accentuated where illness is suffered alone and compounded by the loneliness engendered by prejudice and ignorance. Historically, the expansion of discursive space involving institutions relating to human rights (the 'dignity of man') has always involved the airing of public issues around matters previously invisible to public view, opening up afresh the family or the minority group. This bringing into view – making painful matters public – is an essential part of claims to social justice, and foregrounds issues of visibility for our consideration.

One can see how those who would maintain the *status quo* work to keep knowledge of disease and suffering invisible in the attempt to retain their immunity not only from disease, but from the impact on their scope of action – their values – that an ensuing dialogue must bring. And one way to do this is to keep the disease located within the group, so that it has the character of a tropical disease, one 'proper to a place'. A tropical disease 'only operates *as disease* when it afflicts people from *here*', not there (Patton, 1995: 185 emphasis in original). Applied to the situation of people with AIDS a tropical model says the equivalent of 'I don't live/go there' (Patton, 1995: 189), so that the immunity of the healthy majority is maintained through the domestication and isolation of the group held to be afflicted.

The 'here' and 'there' referred to above are real locations, identifiable with particular groups. This is not the case with discursive/agonistic space, which is defined not by its topography but by forms of action, so that (rather like epidemiology, see Patton (1995)) it has ideological/imaginary form. Protests or sponsored walks involving poster images or markings on the body make space in this way, both discursively and agonistically. They undo the tropicality of disease through the mobility of those afflicted (who might 'invade' areas transgressively) and by making public – by showing forth – those things that the mainstream would keep sequestered to the places occupied by the group (e.g. gay kissing, mastectomy scars). Borrowing, inserting, or traducing mainstream signs are all part of a *theatre of action* that undoes the real by invoking the imaginary. And while speech and persuasion are vital to this, the making of theatre involves tropes (it is *tropical*), making use of mundane features of space, place and material culture to introduce dissonance that provokes inquiry and dialogue.

Where does this leave 'the aesthetic' in relation to social movements that aim to empower ill people, to change public views of disease and to counter media representation of people with AIDS, cancer, or any other disease? First, it shows that aesthetic ways of knowing, of sensing the world and one's place in it can only be understood in relation to the social and political context in which they arise and which they help to create. It is important not to see paintings or photographs as being formative of, or affected by social groupings as if they stood apart from these. Visual depictions constitute material forms in the dialogues that promote and resist the emergence of illness cultures, establishing discursive space related to social practices associated with disease regimes. Representational works are designed for such events and make their sensuous appearance in the course of action; they are open to interpretation afterwards and to subsequent re-interpretation as they are copied, reported or re-exhibited in different contexts. All of this makes them what they are – what they become (Becker, 1982).

This brings us to the point where we can say that a determinist view of artworks as being outside the social context of illness (which influences them), or a constructivist position that regards artworks as needing interpretation in order to bring them into being, are both partly correct yet inadequate. What needs to be recognised is that artworks (or any images making a statement) *in being already ideological,* are constitutive of the illness sphere, working through and on bodies to enable, as far as is possible, their redemptive and emancipatory potential (Radley and Bell, 2007).

Portrayals of Illness as Aesthetic Projects

Although works of illness, produced and deployed individually or collectively, are ideological this is not sufficient reason to explain their impact. Ideology operates through convention, in that meanings are shared and contested about social life in ways that variously legitimate, justify or conflict. The idea of convention carries the implication that works used by activists mean what they do because of established shared meaning. To a large extent this is hardly surprising given how text and visual tropes are designed precisely to subvert mainstream icons. However, artworks – or rather the aesthetic impact of artworks – cannot be reduced to ideological effects. This is because the aesthetic impact is different, even though often coloured by ideology. It is important not to think of ideology and aesthetics as operating quite separately because each may pass through or be reflected in the other. Nevertheless, in their relative superordinacy ideological and aesthetic modes promote and in turn marginalize different aspects of the issues being represented. Pity moved to action produces a collective response, the aim of which is to change the world as part of which suffering and passivity are overcome. In a sense, suffering, if not removed, is transcended through action, removed from its centre as the well-spring of contemplation and, for a while at least, is refused as an identifying condition of those oppressed. To the observer of scenes of activism, the ideological consequence is quite likely a sense of the afflicted being empowered.

Let us use an example to look at this a little closer. The sociologist Catherine Riessman recalled her previous interpretation of a story told to her by a woman who had suffered domestic abuse. The story included an account of domestic rape and of the woman finally throwing her husband out of the house. Riessman reflects upon her reaction to the story some 12 years earlier. She recalls: 'My theoretical and political interest in women's agency shifts the narrative performance. ... I could not let the performance end with a passive heroine resigned to her fate.' (2002: 206). She also remembers that the woman was quite emotional at this point in the story, but that in response, 'as audience, I listen but must look away'. (2002: 207). Riessman's ideological commitment would appear to have led to a partial reading of this woman's story, albeit an important one. What is missing, and what some 12 years later she wants to call back from the margins, is the effect that listening to a horrific story had on the interpretation that she offered – or rather, *had on her*. In the light of her original refusal of an aesthetic response, she recognises the need for researchers to face up to difficult moments of witnessing, even where they are powerless to do anything about them at the time.

In recounting this example I do not want to set ideology against aesthetics but to point up that while activism might employ artistic devices, one of its main purposes is to move beyond pity, and in so doing, to look away from the pitiable. This cannot be a once and only movement because, as already noted, indignation always depends upon keeping in touch with the fate of those on behalf of whom it raises a social voice. (This tension – between the creation of durable institutions that empower the needy as a group and acts of compassion that respond to individual sufferers – is at the heart of all organisations with a charitable aim.) The situation of the ill is not bounded by ideological concerns (though it might be conditioned by them) so that indignation and accusation are not responses that answer all puzzles of suffering. As Boltanski (1999) says, holding in check such emotions makes possible the confrontation of the truth, looking horror in the face. However, as Riessman's story demonstrates, it is not easy to look horror in the face. While not necessarily easier, it is more 'sensible' and 'sensuous' to depict horror by means of practices and performances that employ ascetic distance.

The Subversive Artist: Jo Spence's photo-theatre

One of the first examples of image appropriation by women with breast cancer was the work of the late Jo Spence, a photographer who countered her diagnosis by the visual depiction of her body in health and in illness (Spence, 1988, 1995). In exhibitions, books and workshops she displayed images of her body – often of herself bare-breasted – that challenged the conventional silence about cancer that made its sufferers into invisible victims. On the one hand, she photographed herself in hospital having mammograms and in clinics receiving alternative therapy. On the other, she showed herself – her partly-naked body – in the everyday setting of her home, situating herself on her own ground, in her own context. Using these two kinds of image, she countered the assumption that the female, sick and ageing body is unworthy of visual representation. Also, by showing photographs of her diseased breast she made viewers confront cancer directly, attempting to de-mystify the illness by engaging with the 'horror' of the disease that is central to its invisibility (for background to Spence's work as a photographer see Bell, 2002; Dykstra, 1995; Roberts, 1998). A consideration of Jo Spence's photographs reveals that, while they would later be turned into political icons by the breast cancer movement, they invited, indeed called for, a collective challenge to the hegemony of medicine. This is what was meant earlier, in saying that, in being constitutive of the illness sphere, such works are 'already ideological'.

Jo Spence was an activist who put her art (photography) at the service of her political beliefs. In order to represent her own experience of cancer, she realised that she had to '*become* the documentary object' within her own project (Roberts, 1998: 205). Together with her partner Terry Dennett, she drew upon socialist principles and practice to create images that were intended to further change through consciousness-raising. Her work is deliberately provocative, sometimes transgressive but always challenging and innovative in its use of photographic technique. The two photographs shown here, '*I Framed my Breast for Posterity*' and '*Property of Jo Spence?*' (see Figures 2 and 3) are taken from a set made at the time she was admitted to hospital for possible mastectomy as treatment for her breast cancer.

Spence's photographic work was a response to her sense (accurate at the time) that (a) there was a distressing absence of non-pathological images of breast cancer available, and (b) that there was an under-narrativisation about this disease from the point of view of the women who live with it (Roberts 1998: 205). Finding no images for what she wanted to say, she had to create these out of her own pain and her own imagination, bringing these together through assembling signs where current ideologies of illness and treatment of disease could be contested. Her imagination was rooted in her experience of disease (as we see it on her body) and her pain was given voice in the authorship of the photographic assembly (Scarry 1985). As Roberts (1998) points out, Spence's work was not just an act of bravery or intellectual expediency but was also one of personal and political necessity. This necessity gave rise to a photograph (shown as Figure 2 – '*I Framed my Breast for Posterity*') that marked a turning point in her work, something that Spence recognised at the time (Dennett, 2001). She made the photograph collaboratively with her partner Terry Dennett the night before going into hospital for surgery in 1982. Though it continued their joint work in 'phototheatre' (the fabrication of appearances), this photograph (it was one of three they took that evening) also introduced a new element, 'phototherapy', something that Spence would develop separately. In this context the term 'phototherapy' refers to the way that making work for others has benefits that go beyond what is sometimes thought of as 'making the artist feel better'. Therapy, in this sense, extends to the reconstruction of signs in ways that are in the interests of *all* those who do not traditionally control the production of meanings about illness (see also Gray, et al., 2000). It is less about 'saving one's life' than about 'staying alive' (Spence, 1995: 135).

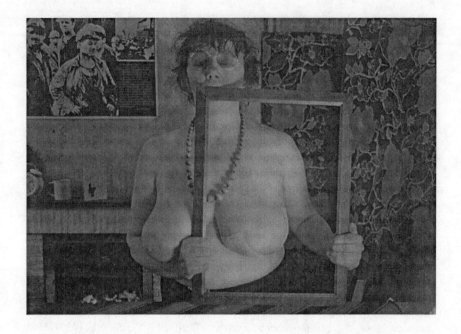

Figure 2. *Jo Spence/Terry Dennett "I Framed my Breast for Posterity", 1982.*
Courtesy of Terry Dennett, The Jo Spence Memorial Archive, London.

To view and to talk about these two photographs is therefore to engage in a co-construction of an ideological position, an approach that Spence deliberately adopted. This is where easily recognisable elements can be juxtaposed in unexpected ways so as to subvert the way that institutions (such as medicine) 'efface their own structures of power within representation' (Spence, 1986: 177). She studied the techniques of the European photographer and socialist John Heartfield, whose work during the inter-war period aimed at critiquing capitalism and totalitarianism. Like Heartfield, Spence turned away form the traditional art gallery as inspiration (though her work was sometimes shown in galleries) towards the world of popular culture and the everyday settings of working class people. She drew upon Heartfield's (and Volosinov's) contention that the sign is primarily the arena of an ideological struggle, and that the re-arrangement of naturalistic signs is an important vehicle for the promotion of a political message.

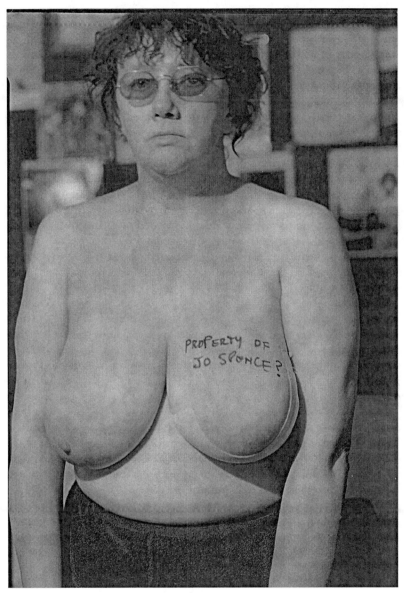

Figure 3. *Jo Spence/Terry Dennett 'Property of Jo Spence?',*
Courtesy of Terry Dennett, The Jo Spence Memorial Archive, London.

Translating this idea into practice, Spence and Dennett adopted what they called 'the intruder technique' in their photographs. This was specifically aimed at disturbance, provocation, rebellion and a witnessing of the shortcomings of medicine within capitalist society (Dennett, 2001). This can be seen in Figure 3, *'Property of Jo Spence?'*, a photograph that was made at the same time. About this picture, Spence (1988: 157) says that this is one of a 'series of tableaux', each with a different caption written on her breast. In this picture she stands, wearing glasses, with her breasts exposed, the writing referring to the site of its inscription. Drawing once more on photography's critical potential, this is an Agitprop shot that, like *'I Framed my Breast for Posterity'*, also draws upon the theatrical.[1] In calling them tableaux, Jo Spence is making clear that these photographs are records of dramaturgical creations that took place, i.e. the photos that one might regard as records of happenings ('visual data') are actually traces of carefully constructed enactments, the form of which the viewer is invited to deconstruct. Or as she and Dennett put it in an account of their working method, 'In this way we have a twin performance; the staging and acting out of a tableau for the camera, and then a two-dimensional signifying performance on paper.' (Spence, 1995: 78).

What photographs like these capture are performances, or what one might call autobiographic portraiture with a history (Dennett, 2001). Unlike portraits that are codified and idealised (as in wedding photography) these images are autobiographical in the sense that they *problematise the relationship between the figure and the artist.* This relationship – which depends upon ascetic distance for its production – initiates a different aesthetic from that of the conventionalised image, but an aesthetic nonetheless. It is one that makes its appearance by 'passing through' the topic of indignation. In this way, to amend Roberts's phrasing, 'photography speaks through the experience of [illness] in order to give social agency to [illness] experience' (1998: 211).

To create the effects in her photographs, Spence used naturalistic items and settings to disrupt, as well as to oppose her material reality to that projected by medicine and the popular media of the time. At base, Jo Spence's pictured breasts are a counter to both medicalised breasts (the 'sick' versus the 'healthy' breast) and to breasts that are revealed in the glamour press. There is, as Roberts (1998: 210) has pointed out, an *anti-aestheticism* in

---

[1] 'Property of Jo Spence' is also a documentary photo, although staged – shot as a record of the text to remind the hospital staff that this was the cancer affected breast – a documentary photo to take into hospital with her (p.c. Dennett, 2006).

Spence's work, especially in the picture *Property of Jo Spence?*. The use of text is an acknowledgment of the inability to picture illness experience, and a refusal to offer images that either borrow from or could be returned to the world of consumer culture. Unlike the ACT UP icons, or even the pictures in the 'Obsessed with Breasts' campaign, the ordinariness of Spence's props stand in the way of their being appropriated stylistically. They offer instead a basis for shared experience, a placing of her world on to which other women – those from the British working class, or with bodies similar to hers – could map their own experience.

While the juxtaposition of signs allows for the production of powerful images, it is important not to read Spence's later accounts of struggle at the personal level as diminishing the claim that her pictures were ideological in design. From their moments of creation they invited a viewing (and reading) that is simultaneously personal as well as social and political. Spence was struggling to be heard by her surgeon so she could get the treatment she believed she needed. She was also struggling to be heard by other women, so that her experiences could be useful to them. She wanted them to know that they, like she, could think and act differently about breast cancer. As was the case with her earlier political work, she wanted to help create a community, this time a community of 'dissident cancer patients' (Spence, 1995: 214).

Becoming an Activist through Art

The use of naturalistic items in Spence's work echoes the mundane features of the lives of some (but not all) of the women who will look at them. This is true both for tableaux pictures and for photographs that were clearly of documentary form. The photographs taken during her time in hospital depict an alien environment – medical technology – to which some viewers of her pictures might relate. The transformation of the mundane – whether to interrupt or otherwise – is a common feature of work that elicits an aesthetic response. It poses alternative ways of looking and challenges conventional ways of understanding. It is by virtue of this transformation of the material world that artist and viewer find themselves refigured in the cycle of creation and consumption. In their initial stages, which will come to be seen as a re-framing, such photographs have the feel of documentary in the collection and re-assembly of material. Spence described how her work on picturing health had two roots: one in the earlier work she had carried out on deconstructing images of the family, and the other in the 'banal snapshots' of herself she had available. Placing these snapshots against details of her health and treatment she decided to 'visually document my struggle for health', and to see how that might be allied to campaigns in other fields, notably anti-nuclear campaigns (Spence, 1988: 155). What is interesting is how, from its inception, this work is energised by indignation, moved by compassion (care for self and others) and directed by an ascetic intelligence that guides this apparently simple re-assembly of times, details of disease and personal portraiture.

We can see a very similar occurrence in the account given by Martha Hall, an American maker of artist's books, talking about her work as a medium for communicating her experience of being a woman with breast cancer (for an overview of Hall's work, see Bell, 2006). Martha Hall did not share Jo Spence's working class background, but she did share something of the experience of being diagnosed with breast cancer even though (unlike Spence) she opted for mastectomy and associated medical treatment. Diagnosed with breast cancer in 1989, she began making artist's books in 1993, completing her first in 1996 and going on to make over 100 of these until her death in December 2003. The medium she worked in is interesting from the point of view of re-assembling mundane elements of life to make art.

The artist's book has been described as an emergent form of the 20th century: 'It is a zone made at the intersection of a number of different disciplines, fields, and ideas – rather than at their limits ' (Drucker (1995: 1, para 2). Unlike the illustrated book, artist's books use the book form as a flexible format to interweave text with symbol in a plurality of 'textilities'. For example, one of Martha Hall's books – titled '*Just to Live*' – is described in the exhibition catalogue as being made of 'mixed media collage: cloth, photo Xerox, metal, medical tubing, stitching, rice paper, paste paper, postage stamps. Altered envelopes, medical tests and films, watercolour inkjet and handwritten in coloured ink (Hall, 2003: 89). What is striking in this description – what is interruptive – is the combination of forms and textures, brought together in a single artefact. It is impossible to reproduce Hall's artist's books here, except to indicate with photographs what her books look like from the outside. This inability to make multiple copies of her work is important, not just because it limits its exposure but because it highlights a different way of opening a collective, discursive space in which ideologies of illness can first be brought into the open, and then challenged.

Another of her books – *The Rest of My Life* – parallels Spence's description of re-assembly in being made up of her medical appointment cards, so that the book is of this size. The cards span a year's chemotherapy appointments, are completed in the same hand, are put together with surgical tape and bandages and between some of the cards are pill packages some containing pills. Describing what it is like to handle this book, Susan Bell says:

The book opens like a long two-sided accordion, to 64 inches. On one side, the appointment cards are pink, printed with the words, "Maine Center for Cancer Medicine & Blood Disorder;" turn the cards over and there is a white background, printed with the Cancer Center's address and telephone number, and spaces to be filled in with a patient's (given) name, day of the week, date, and time of the appointment. ... All of them have been "used." The book is contained in a small box, itself covered with Hall's appointment calendar for October 1999.

On the back of the cards are several layers of handwritten text by Hall in different colors of ink and different styles of handwriting. In brown ink there is a timeline from 1989 when Hall discovered a lump in her left breast to the present, 2000. This layer of text is printed, neatly. Another layer of text, in black ink cursive, records questions and answers between her and other patients and friends, and an internal dialogue ... (Bell, 2006).

What could be more apposite as an exemplar of life made into art than this 'book' – which is more than a book? It brings together in a new way – not just interrupting but re-juxtaposing – mundane elements drawn from Martha Hall's experience of medical treatment. This allows readers to be taken along with her, 'as they see the same loopy handwriting filling in the cards over and over, each time for "Martha" and each time for a different date; and they can hold the same cards and the same pill packages that Martha held, first as a breast cancer patient, and then as an artist.' (Bell, 2006). (I have not held this book, but the image of that 'loopy handwriting', appearing in Martha Hall's mailbox each month, drawing her back to the clinic, sends a shiver down my spine.)

The photographs made by Spence (with Dennett) and the artist's books made by Hall are works of illness in the sense that they problematise not only the individual's relationship to her illness, but also her relationship to the world of health and its institutionalised treatment practices. What energises the aesthetic is indignation, a feeling not vaporised in the artistic endeavour but rather transformed through trope and metaphor into forms that speak afresh about the alterity of ill people. That sense of solidarity with other women who suffer breast cancer does not spring forth ready made, a coherent precursor to the fabrication of the work itself. While Jo Spence (1988) tells of her working class upbringing and her disillusion with the world of professional photography, it was in the course of her work with other radical artists and with other students of photography that she gave her political outrage an aesthetic dimension.

Within a very different background – but leading to a similar set of practices – Martha Hall re-discovered her indignation in the course of an artist's workshop. This was a 'transformative event', a critical moment in which she could see that she had to share her experiences with others and that she must do this by means of expressive forms that she could control – making art. In a rare testimony to the role of the mundane as supportive of social difference, and hence similarity, she made a work that shows its own rationale.

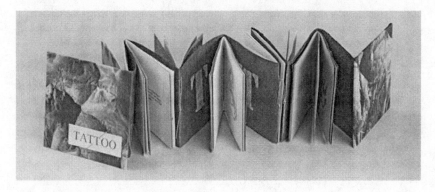

Figure 4. *Martha Hall, "Tattoo", 1998. 4 3/8 x 4 3/8 x 1 inches, opens to 32 inches. Photograph by Dennis Griggs, Courtesy the George J. Mitchell Department of Special Collections & Archives, Bowdoin College Library, Brunswick, Maine.*

Figure 4 shows a picture of *Tattoo*, a small square book, made of coloured papers, printed and paste paper and boards, that opens like a double-sided accordion, to 32". It contains eight short stories written by Hall, each printed and illustrated with a simple rubber stamp or stencil. The cover is printed with coloured paper, in blue, black, and a bit of white. The linearity of this artist's book is deceptive, because it is a reconstruction narrative that retains the breaks in Hall's life wrought by her cancer. In eight stanzas (or stories) she sets out how she came to feel the need to speak out to other women about her cancer, and how this was premised upon recognition of difference. The sign that she deploys in different ways is the tattoo marks made on the breast (or elsewhere on the body) to aid in the administration of radiotherapy. The title, *Tattoo*, signals something, perhaps unfamiliar to outsiders, about the medical world of (breast) cancer. Tattoos carry a message about the social and feminist world of breast cancer. Some women have chosen to mark themselves with tattoos after surgery for breast cancer. These tattoos become part of 'the palimpsest of breast cancer' that is written on their bodies (Langellier, 2001:145). A sewing needle is stuck into the cover of *Tattoo*, much as a needle might be temporarily stored when a sewing project is underway. This is not a needle that would be used in a tattoo parlour. But as a sewing needle it connects the art of book-making to the activities of sewing and cloth making. The sewing needle also echoes the tattoo's 'stereotypic and stigmatising associations,' in its suggestion of a makeshift tool for marking the body (Langellier, 2001:147). For Hall in her younger (healthy) days, tattoos were marks of otherness, of transgression. They signified things outside her white middle-class upbringing, something that made identification with women in general difficult, and also her acceptance of ideologies that kept her a passive victim of her disease.

At the physical turning of *Tattoo* Hall tells of an encounter through which she realizes that she must share her experiences of breast cancer with others. (At this point, the book must be turned over, so that the viewer/reader must *make the turn with Hall*, as she goes 'from one side to the other'.) This formative experience happens at an artist's workshop. Hall's telling of this story begins with an all-too-familiar rehearsal of racial prejudice and homophobia, subsequently subverted by the man's actions and words.[2]

> This summer at Haystack I shared a
> studio table with George from
> Philadelphia,
> a very tall black man with a shaved
> head
> who made complex, powerful,
> angry art.
> He was loud, brash, gay.
> I was afraid of him –
> Then I heard him sing in a beautiful

---

[2] Hall's initial response to this man recapitulates a certain way in which white people "look" at black people: through an "imperial eye" that sees "the black subject as a marauding native, menacing savage or rebellious slave" (Mercer, 1994: 178). Perhaps one could argue that because 'Curious George' is a monkey, taken from the jungle by the Man in the Yellow Hat (in the first book in the Curious George series), the juxtaposition of Curious George merely exemplifies a "bifurcation in racial representations," the imperial eye, an unstated but nonetheless potent racialized representation of George from Philadelphia (Mercer, 1994: 178; Rey, 1973).

soprano voice as he worked
and saw that the tattoo on his
muscular brown arm was

Curious George.

One night he looked at the book I
was making
called 'Living'
and told me that when he was sixteen
his mother had died of breast cancer.[3]

'Curious George' is a friendly monkey in an American picture book series, known to generations of children and parents (Rey, 1973). Hall writes about this meeting again in the "Artist's Statement" for the catalogue of her exhibition *Holding In, Holding On* (Hall, 2003). What she was holding in, she tells us, were her feelings, until she realised that she needed to share them with others. This realisation is made possible by what the man said to her concerning the time of his mother's death, words that do not appear in *Tattoo* itself. He said, simply "I wish I had thought to make art about it then" (Hall, 2003: 12).

The story-in-the-story is worth repeating here on two counts. First, it is exemplary of how visual images – in this instance tattoo marks – can become anchoring points. Second, the way it is told (*with the book* itself, something it is not possible to reproduce here) displays – re-presents for readers – the arrangement of signifiers that was disruptive of Hall's experience that day. The disruption comes from the unusual (for Hall) conjunction and contextualisation of signs in her meeting with the man, whose 'transgressive' features (his blackness, very tall size, being gay) were juxtaposed with his artistic ability, his beautiful voice, and his 'Curious George' tattoo. By the end of the meeting these signs have undergone a curious inversion, so that Hall now identifies herself with the transgressive, with the man who felt he should have 'spoken out' about breast cancer.

This unexpected juxtaposition of easily recognisable elements (spontaneous in the meeting, crafted in the artist's book) is reminiscent of the conditions that Spence (1986) set out deliberately to reconstruct in her photographs. In both cases signifiers are re-presented so as to present afresh an ideological challenge to the *status quo*. It is in the re-arrangement of signs that Hall recognises herself as being more than a woman with breast cancer,

---

[3] This is the fourth story in Tattoo.

but also a person with a responsibility to share her experiences with others through her art. The signs that are there in her meeting with the man are re-framed by the story he tells about his own mother's cancer, a characterisation in which, we argue, she recognises something of her own situation. The role of 'mother' is important to Hall, sufficiently so that she begins her artist's statement in the exhibition catalogue with the words 'The day before Mother's Day, 1989…a surgeon I did not know phoned me …' (Hall 2003:10). This sign vehicle is important to aid in the recognition of another similarity, this time with the man's past failure to speak out on behalf of his mother and people like her (like Hall). This apprehension of a moment from the past in the sign constellation of the present figures her own sense of duty to speak out, and with that a radical transformation of the meaning of being the sort of person who has made, or makes upon themselves, a tattoo. What Hall makes of this is a re identification of herself as an artist with breast cancer, a person with a message and a means to communicate it to others.

Ideology and Interpretation

I want to conclude this chapter with a brief discussion of the role of ideology in the interpretation of artworks, particularly the kind of visual works that have been discussed so far. Earlier on, I asked the questions, 'what is the relationship of the aesthetic and political dimensions within works of illness?', and 'how might one overshadow the other?' The answers to these questions rest upon a recognition that such works do not come either before or after their political and social deployment. Rather, we need to see them as being both ways of articulating ideas and, in their public appearance, as nodal points around which people can assemble. They are part of material culture and the culture of activism to which they belong, and so are inadequately understood if taken merely as reflections of ideology or as stimuli to action. This is not to detract from the role of ideology in their fabrication, nor is it to draw attention from the fact that some artworks become iconic in the course of being identified with a movement or cause.

This means that works of illness are not reducible *either* to their aesthetic *or* to their political dimensions. Being produced in the crucible of indignation, with compassion for fellow sufferers, and by virtue of techniques at the artist's disposal, these works are made to signify in multiple ways. It is therefore not surprising that they can be interpreted – or particular meanings drawn out and amplified – depending upon context and the purposes to which they are directed. This raises the further question whether we need to be able to interpret the ideological significance of a painting or photograph to understand it. There is the danger here that one takes the object of interpretation – the 'it' – to be the picture in itself, when we know that the kinds of works described in this chapter were created precisely to promote inquiry and dialogue about matters in the world beyond the frame, over which they have virtual control (to which they imaginatively refer). Having said that, it would be a mistake to say, for example, that Spence's photograph '*I Framed My Breast For Posterity*' is understood first from knowledge of the British class system and the hegemony of medicine. We do not interpret first and then see after. The references made to the mundane, and to the transposition of naturalistic elements across different spheres or within the one artefact, point to the way in which these act as points of recognition in our viewing. This recognition is not in itself value free, but it is subject in its everyday aspect to an aesthetic of its own – an erotic – that we should do well to remember. The ordinary is not without its own charge, linked with desire and with repugnance. Those things that are disturbing, frightening or horrific can also be fascinating and tempting to the eye. When Jo Spence displays herself naked from the waist up the viewer is subject to a transgressive gaze that undoes a comfortable viewing. The viewer of such works has already entered into a spontaneous interpretation but along paths of similarity and of desire/repugnance in which they find themselves already engaged.

In the case of Spence's images, the 'phototheatre' to which she refers is not limited to a time when the picture was made, but appears again now in the agonistic space – the space of theatre – that her picture creates for the viewer, alongside the depicted 'interruptions' that promote a discursive response. This means that no matter how conventionalised a picture might become in its adoption by a social movement, its potential as a work (its erotic charge) is always there to be grasped along with its ideological message. And no matter the efforts made to remove a painting or photograph from the everyday world of politics, the ideological interests of viewers will find connections with apparently mundane elements and with conventions of representation to enable dialogue to be opened. In relation to the double movement of the aesthetic and the ideological, pictures and stories enter into and are in turn penetrated by a changing world of illness and its treatment. There can be no closure here, so that while the meaning accorded to works of illness is indeterminate, their potential remains really quite considerable.

Chapter 3

'Making present' for Others:
the art of witness

Any discussion of pictures and stories in the context of activism assumes a particular kind of relationship between the outraged or dispossessed and others who are potential supporters of their position. However, not all representations of illness are made from, or exist wholly within, the frame of activism. There are those who see pictures or read stories to do with illness for whom the making public of suffering is not primarily a call to action. Amongst these are individuals who read stories or gaze at pictures in a spirit of consumption. And there are those who, faced with these texts and pictures, simply turn away. Ours is a time when care and concern for the public realm cannot be assumed as a matter of course. There are people for whom freedom *from* the public realm has supplanted freedom within it. A life of looking and looking away – where the afflicted are objectified in their distant condition – is characteristic of a specular engagement that leads to a peculiar 'reduction of corporeality to the eye' (Tester, 1997: 75). This specular relationship has, as one of its key characteristics, being 'aesthetic' – but now in the sense of alienation produced by the very instruments that bring the image/text closer to us. It was this kind of image and story that was criticised by activists concerned at the photographs taken of people with AIDS. Critics saw these pictures as confirming the observer as someone who looks upon a person with AIDS as being in the position of victim. This gives rise to an ongoing concern with the moral sensitivity that people have with respect to images of suffering in the world, to ideas of 'compassion fatigue' and the possible deadening of our sensibilities as a result of the steady drip of horrendous images seen via television and the Internet.

In her essay on photography, Sontag (1979) argued that one of the leading tendencies in modern art has been that of suppressing or reducing moral and sensory queasiness. By this she meant that we are encouraged to get used to seeing what we cannot bear to see, urged not to be upset but 'to confront the horrible with equanimity' (1979: 41). She concluded that, despite the illusion of providing understanding, photography instead homogenises and anaesthetises; it promotes, through aesthetic awareness, an emotional detachment. Put this way, the visual depiction of illness is at odds with attempts to change the situation of those who are sick. It gives rise to an observer who – given a sufficient flow of images – watches, if not without sentiment, then without commitment. This implies a gaze with which we are familiar in the modern metropolis; the look of the blasé (Simmel, 1968), the *flâneur* (Benjamin, 1970) and the glimpses of each other with which we satisfy ourselves in public places (Goffman, 1976). This should not be seen merely as a function of the sensibilities of the modern individual. The Western media work so as to appropriate 'the cultural capital of trauma victims – their wounds, their scars, their tragedy – [using] the same popular codes through which physical and sexual violence are commodified, sold in the cinema, marketed as pornography, and used by tabloids and novelists to attract readers' (Kleinman and Kleinman, 1997: 10-11). And yet in spite of this, the capacity of images to affect people – perhaps some people, at some times – is not eradicated, as Sontag (2003) herself was later to admit. I was struck by this fact when carrying out research into charitable giving, finding that individuals (not the exception) would respond strongly to photographs related to a disease condition from which a family member had suffered and perhaps died (Radley and Kennedy, 1997). Even with respect to photographs of thin and ailing babies in Africa, thought to have become a staple of the charity industry, I have seen a woman respondent reduced to tears. Perhaps in these cases the pictures touched something in the lives of those respondents, attesting to realities that these photographs confirmed rather than elided, so to speak. Certainly where disease and illness strike near to home, stories and pictures take on a significance that belies talk of 'compassion fatigue'.

The role of artworks in the creation of the public realm, and their appearances within and outside of it, is therefore important but not exclusive in the making of aesthetic responses to illness and its treatment. In fact, a key justification for the study of illness narratives in the social sciences has been that these stories provide interesting and important *insights* into the illness condition. It is arguable that the social sciences have, so far, been less concerned with the political role of these and other works (especially visual representations) than have people in the arts in general, for whom the reception of their works is always contestable. Being scientists of a sort, sociologists addressing health issues have been more concerned with epistemological matters, concerned with the validity of stories (they have hardly touched on visual works) as evidence of the illness condition. However, scientific, juridical or specular issues do not exhaust the question of how people respond to works addressing the world of the seriously ill. This is because there is an aesthetic that arises in the relationship between artists/writers and individuals who are ready and willing to engage with the work in its singularity. I speak of 'an aesthetic' here to distinguish this topic from the 'aesthetics of activism', or the 'aesthetics of consumption', the latter drawing upon the distance between life and art that a modernist view permits.

This other position might be called 'the aesthetic of witness' in order to emphasise that its rationale lies in a confirmation by the reader or viewer of a semblance of illness that the work is able to show forth. This idea of semblance distinguishes this way of showing from the documentary, be it in narrative or photographic form. It is not a more distinct and public confirmation of the real that is proposed in such works, but something nearer to the sublime in the sense of conveying what, even if it cannot be seen, might yet be touched. The test of such affirmations then resides in ideas-with-feeling evoked in the reader or viewer, for whom the work illuminates something previously in shadow, or names something that was previously inchoate. This might or might not relate to shared experiences, but where it does – as when Jo Spence described women with breast cancer who saw her photographs as 'falling about her with open arms' – then the meaning of the work is confirmed in the response of the reader or viewer. The meaning of such stories or paintings is intimately tied up with the work they do for others, but internally, so to speak. Where the aesthetic of activism is shaped in its commerce with politics, the testing or the movement of boundaries between groups, an *agonistic* aesthetic is associated with a dissolving of boundaries between individuals. To the extent that stories, plays, paintings and photographs evoke a mutual recognition of travails, suffering or coping in the face of adversity, then they do this kind of work. Authors and artists feel their voice not only heard but also recognised. Readers and viewers say that they sense the fulfilment of some need, or the validation of illness experience that until then had made them feel both isolated and silenced. An important aspect of this response is the sense that something has been given to the reader or the viewer by the work, that there is a kind of gift involved. What is this gift; how is it made, and what are the conditions for speaking in these terms about a work that, to all intents and purposes, might have been appropriated as a commodity in the form of a book or a photograph seen in a commercial gallery?

The Space of Interiority: compassion and the illness question

We need to pick up again Hannah Arendt's distinction between compassion and pity, which she saw as distinguishable in their relation to generalisable forms, and hence to politics (Arendt, 1973). Compassion is the immediate sense of another's suffering which issues in a practical response; it is linked to *presence* and it implies a practical engagement with the 'horrors' that accompany mortal decline. (The parable of the Good Samaritan is a good illustration of this condition, which locates it firmly in the Christian tradition of Western societies.) By comparison, pity is a different response, conditional upon the secularization of philanthropy, something that operates on the basis of a generalization of suffering, as to the poor, or the sick, or another class of individuals. As we have seen, pity has an essentially political dimension in its distancing of the observer from the sufferer. This distancing is crucial in setting up the 'durable institutions' needed to organise a social response, as part of which, in the modern world, is the attempt to establish equal rights that will overturn a 'pitiable' response. Paradoxically, in a world of rights and justice, the word 'pity' carries negative overtones. This is not true for compassion, because to lack compassion is to be without feeling, and therefore to risk moral condemnation. That is why activism must return to, or repeatedly re-engage with compassion in order to demonstrate a caring attitude to those who suffer or who cannot improve their situation. Stories and artworks deployed in the name of indignation actually presume the 'pity' that they strive to surpass. They articulate difference and objectify anger through helping to create spatial and temporal distance. By comparison, says

Arendt, compassion is mute in its response, conveyed immediately through action to relieve suffering, so that:

> For compassion to be stricken with the suffering of someone else as
> though it were contagious, and pity, to be sorry without being touched in
> the flesh, are not only not the same *but they may not even be related.*
> Compassion, by its very nature, cannot be touched off by the sufferings
> of a whole class of people, or, least of all, mankind as a whole. It cannot
> reach out farther than what is suffered by one person and still remain
> what it is supposed to be, co-suffering. (1973: 85, emphasis added).

I read this as saying that compassion and pity have different roots, not that they are unrelated in the efforts of people to relieve suffering. What is important for an analysis of aesthetic responses to illness experience is that compassion be recognised as involving the *presence* of individuals, being touched '*in the flesh*', and the *co-suffering* of those concerned. Regarding the way that images or stories of illness work in this regard, it is not the conditions for the appearance of compassion in general in which we are interested, but the potential of works of illness to fabricate those conditions for others. The question then becomes one of describing the ways that stories and pictures mediate or express illness so that a compassionate response becomes possible. This includes not only the response of fellow sufferers, but also that of individuals who feel with or for the afflicted person. And whereas, in 'activist art', works are aimed at re-positioning individuals and groups, the 'art of compassion' has the aim of *creating presence, touching the reader or viewer in the flesh*, and *establishing co-suffering* between one who gives and one who receives. While it is not possible to draw clear lines of demarcation between illness situations and their respective forms of response, it would seem that compassion is elicited in situations where indignation is either deemed inappropriate or does not arise. It might be that individuals do not see their situation as the responsibility of others, but regard a serious illness as a matter of fate that they must bear without rancour. And in cases of extreme suffering the urgency of gesture and appeal is such that a compassionate response is demanded, and granted, in advance (if not in exclusion) of the mobilisation of social action.

Whatever the case, the accompanying sentiment to compassion is tender heartedness, not indignation. As such it has what Boltanski (1999) calls its own metaphysics, a metaphysics of interiority. This requires that the unfortunate's suffering be confirmed in terms of the reader's or viewer's own response, at the level of the heart. To be touched 'in the flesh' by suffering that is in one's presence is the corollary to being affected in a shudder by the horror of illness making its appearance. Boltanski argues that this is integral with the formation of a relationship between the afflicted person and the other, something that allows the latter to share with others the emotion that touched him or her. This establishes a collectivity, not through a convergence of judgement but through an 'emotional contagion' passing as it were from interior to interior. This requires the creation of presence, and the effective revelation of feeling so that when the reader or viewer 'opens his heart to accept the trace left by suffering' of the afflicted person, this is experienced as a moment of emotion and truth. That truth, says Boltanski, is manifestation. This truth cannot be established in a world of objects and rules because,

> It is not inscribed within the world like a text, which is available to everyone through a reading, interpretation or decoding. It is only ever by making the detour through one's own interiority, by following *the route of the heart*, that one can put oneself in the presence of an interiority, which manifests itself. (Boltanski, 1999: 82, emphasis in original).

How can compassion be conveyed and the sentiment of tender heartedness be experienced? This touching presence, the evocation of urgency, is most easily recognised in the use of the body in expressionist gesture, where the truth of suffering is established by its manifestation with the body in the presence of the other. Here we are in the realm of tears and anguish. However, the reality of feeling is not located at the level of the body's expressions but is referred inside – to the heart – so that its significance lies not in tests of its objective validity, but in the veracity of its manifestation. This applies equally to representations of suffering as to suffering *in vivo*, where in the former case the plane of expression is not with the body but on the canvas, or in print or on the stage. The shedding of tears in weeping is phenomenally different from that in crying, which Koestler (1964) associated with the 'self-assertive emotions' such as anger or fear. By comparison, to weep is to realise what Koestler called participatory or self-transcending emotion. These feelings cannot be satisfied through action but tend towards quiescence, tranquillity and catharsis. He identified these feelings with raptness, the welling-up of feeling, in which the relationship (to a loved one, a piece of music) is embodied, literally, in the living through of the experience.

The metaphysics of interiority involves, as far as aesthetics is concerned, not only a particular kind of response involving co-sufferers, but also a special kind of work done by the mediation, be it a photograph, stage play or story. For example, rather than emphasise actions and decisions in a sequence, the sentiment in a story like *Uncle Tom's Cabin* (which can appear naïve and 'corny' to the modern reader) is 'known by the sound of a voice, the touch of a hand, but chiefly in moments of greatest importance, by tears' (Tompkins, 1985: 131).[4] Tompkins argues that the truths that Stowe's narrative conveys 'can only be re-embodied', which we can take to mean communicated by virtue of the re-placing of features, one with another. To examine this further we need to look at some examples of works that raise questions about the limiting conditions under which certain kinds of aesthetic response are called out. In particular, we need to distinguish, at this point, the special response to artists/authors *and* their works from the response to suffering in general.

Conditions of Authorship

The special conditions we need to examine are those attaching to works that are made by people suffering from illness, in comparison to those made about them by others. The reason for this is that stories and pictures made by sufferers are those that keep us firmly in the grey area that is 'art for illness's sake', the sphere whose locus if not its legitimacy is so often placed in question. For example, Figure 5 shows a picture titled *Self-portrait with Dr Arrieta*, in which Francisco Goya depicted himself seriously ill in bed, being supported by his doctor who is shown offering him a life-saving medicine. He inscribed the painting 'Goya thankful to his friend Arrieta: for the skill and care with which he saved his life during his short and dangerous illness, endured at the end of 1819, at seventy three years of age' (Tomlinson, 1994). In this picture Goya portrays himself as conscious, possibly near to death, but complicit with his doctor in the efforts of medicine to overcome disease. It is a testimony to the success of medical care and an expression of the gratitude of the patient that was forthcoming. Indeed, one might say that this painting is one that elicits compassion only through it being met in the ministrations of the doctor. While it is an autobiographical painting, the subject of the work is less Goya's suffering than the expertise of medicine in the person of Arrieta. This painting bears direct comparison with a more recent work by the late Robert Pope, who was treated for Hodgkin's Disease in Toronto in the 1980s (Murray, 1994). This is one of a number of drawings and paintings that he made as a result of this experience and which form a permanent exhibition (Pope, 1991). Figure 6 titled *Self-Portrait with Dr Langley* shows his doctor in the act of feeling the lymph nodes in Pope's neck, to check the

---

[4] I am grateful to David Morris for pointing me to this observation.

progress of his cancer. Pope says that he tried to draw his own face so as to convey the question, 'has the cancer recurred?'. Unlike in Goya's painting, the relationship between doctor and patient in Pope's drawing is shown – and explained – to be one in which the patient's experience is of paramount importance. Both pictures are autographic in the sense that each depicts the artist in question; and yet Pope's drawing opens up ethical questions that the fatality of Goya's painting does not.

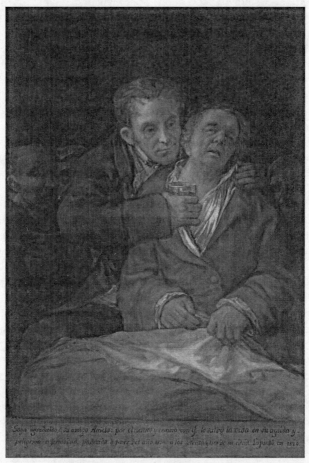

Figure 5. *Francisco Jose de Goya y Lucientes,*
"Self-Portrait with Dr Arrieta", 1820. 137.16 x 99.38 x 9.53 cm (F),
Courtesy Minneapolis Institute of Arts, The Ethel Morrison Van Derlip Fund.

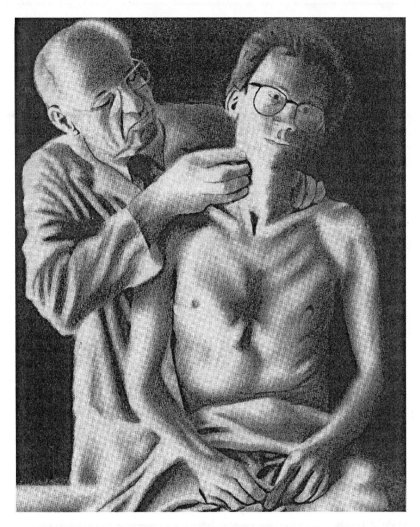

Figure 6. *Robert Pope, "Self-portrait with Dr Langley", 1990. Charcoal on paper, 40.6 x 33.4 cm. Courtesy of the Robert Pope Foundation, Hantsport, Nova Scotia.*

The relatively modern genre of illness narratives is virtually defined by the autopathography, to borrow a term coined by Couser (1997). The autobiographical account depends for its impact – if that is the correct word – upon the way that the author presents herself or himself as a screen through which the horrors of serious illness may be pictured. What emerges from such accounts is not just a story of disease, its treatment and the vicissitudes of recovery, but the way that the author coped with both illness and the discomforts of treatment. The narrative form, with its plots and discursive strategies makes self-reference not only extant but integral with the story. It is in no small measure the assumed correspondence between author and figure that encourages the reader to judge the validity of the account in terms of affirmations of feeling that are put forward in the text. Merely to affirm that 'this happened to me' may be insufficient if what is inchoate about illness is to be indicated. Something in excess of the story as a series of events, or even as a plot, must be expressed. This is reflected in the writing, in *how* the story is put together, so as to conjure a sense of what it is like to face (and bear) the rigours of serious disease. The successful deployment of narrative skills brings about the construction of a screen that not only names illness, but also figures the writer as someone who appears differently in the light of their having coped with the horror of disease.

For Frank, quoting Gabriel Marcel, the correspondence between author and figure on which validity relies is enabled by the claim that, 'We are concerned with a certainty which I *am* rather than with a certainty which I have', (1995: 140, emphasis in original). This idea underlines the claim that a key feature of 'works of illness' is their presentational form, so that while other people might have the story, only the person herself can be it. 'The proof of this testimony is that the witnesses *are* what they testify' (Frank, 1995: 140, emphasis in original). Such testimony demands that testimony be seen, and seen not just on but *with* the body of the person concerned. This points to a distinction between, on the one hand, witnessing suffering, and on the other hand *bearing* witness to suffering. It is not essential that sufferer and witness always be the same person, as is the case in stories or pictures made about people in pain or in need. There are compassionate stories by artists and writers aplenty, including Thomas Mann and Tolstoy. What is different in the case of many 'works of illness' is that they are autobiographical, and that this condition is of paramount importance in their function and significance. What needs to be 'seen' is not the mask of horror, certainly not 'suffering itself'. It is the act of witnessing that must be made manifest, an integral part of which is the authenticity of its biography. Frank makes the point that in contrast to testimony in a traffic court where a written deposition might suffice, in the case of illness the witness (the sufferer) must be seen as a 'whole body'. In saying this he alludes to the special condition that defines autopathography, to use Couser's term once again: works of illness do not merely denote what suffering is like, nor do they just provide a diary-like account of the illness experience. Rather, they are *infra-referential* in their way of narrating or picturing (Latour, 1988). Only in this way can they create the conditions under which the viewer or reader can be touched by the experience denoted, and recognise the author/artist for what they are or have become.

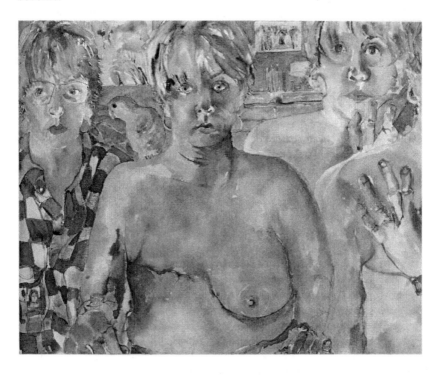

Figure 7. *Elissa Hugens Aleshire, "Self-Portrait", 1998. Image from* Art.Rage.Us: The Art and Outrage of Breast Cancer, *Courtesy the Breast Cancer Fund. www.breastcancerfund.org*

To explain this further, we can look at the self-portrait by Elissa Aleshire (Figure 7) in which she shows herself to us as she sees herself in the mirror after her mastectomy. Looking at the figures in this picture, it soon becomes clear that the figures shown are steps in working up to the painting itself, a record of the path taken prior to her feeling able to pick up the brush, to remove her clothing and stand before the mirror. This is not a work just of the moment, but a record of a passage, by which we are led along with her towards what is difficult and painful to look at. To call this painting a self-portrait is true, but somehow insufficient. It is self-referential in being more than a likeness; it is also a narrative of recovery, of what is effectively an act of self-repossession. As part of this, the signature on a painting or the identification of the person as 'this particular individual' is important in the establishment of the person's suffering and ways of coping with it. And yet, we must not confuse the *person* who is denoted by the picture with the *figure* who is both denoted and expressively presented within it.

It is important to recognise that, in being artefacts that are 'allowed to remain in the made-up stage' (Scarry, 1985: 311), works of art display what she called 'the productive arc' of their fabrication. Part of *being a work* is the announcement of its unique identity, so that the signature of a portrait is in the totality of its expressive form, not just in the signed name of the artist at the foot of the painting or alongside the photograph. (This is, of course, what makes necessary and possible the verification of authenticity of works of art in the modern world). As Scarry emphasises, the 'madeness' of a work of art is not simply recognised and recoverable but it is *self-announcing* and it is this that both celebrates and makes possible the nature of its creation. It is through the apprehension of this creation that we see in the portrait the signature of the sufferer figured, who is 'self-possessed' by the individual denoted. In a self-portrait such as that by Elissa Aleshire, the expressive qualities that are exemplified by the figure are attributed by the observer to Aleshire as a person. This situation is common to all forms of body art that use visual depiction, where the observer sees a person instantiated in his or her portrayal. The perception of the figural qualities of the work denoted by the artist as being of a 'self' is in one sense an illusion, and yet is the condition for our perception of the picture as 'real', or even as 'true'. This is not to say that the portrait of 'suffering-as-borne' is intended primarily as a disclosure of 'self' or feeling. Rather, the self-as-model is the material basis by virtue of which the world of 'illness-as-borne' can be conjured.

This condition, that works (of art, of illness) be self-announcing, is key to the idea put forward by Frank that the ill person wants to be seen not only 'in' but 'as' the story. For people who have undergone extreme suffering, testifying in this way – by means of speech, text or paint – is not a distillation of knowledge but knowing oneself again *only* through making testimony. The knowledge of what one went through – something that cannot be named or delineated – is not of a residual form that can be separated out and communicated as information. Rather, the knowledge that the witness brings *happens* in the *act* of testifying, through the making of a work, so that, 'in its performative aspect, the testimony … can be thought of as a sort of signature' (Felman, 1995: 53).

Clearly then, it is insufficient to define this form of self-reference in terms of denotation: most autobiographies contain the pronoun 'I' but this does not guarantee this kind of signature. Rather, it is the appearance of the work as an exemplar of how to live through illness that is important, so that to grasp that ethic is to grasp the (figured) person as well. All paintings and poems are self-referential in that sense, even where their subject matter is about other people or other things, animate or inanimate. Only a small number of Robert Pope's (1991) pictures of patients, staff, friends and family in the hospital setting include self-portraits, yet all are self-contained works that convey something of suffering and care (see also Figure 16, p. 173). That, in many cases, the persons drawn are unknown to the viewer – are indeed imaginary figures – does not detract in any way from their expressive function. They attest to what Pope saw and what he experienced. And taken as a set of drawings and paintings, the style of rendering is autographic of his way of handling the materials, so it is principally as artist (not as sufferer) that he appears in his work. The word 'principally' points to the fact that, for the reader who is told of Pope's illness and the time he spent in hospital, he comes to appear as both through his work. Even this, however, guarantees no specific compassionate response should the particular drawing or painting fail to be seen as 'effectively' expressing care or suffering. The knowledge that Pope was seriously ill matters when looking at his pictures, but this knowledge alone cannot make them expressive works. That they are composed with artistic skill – with ascetic distance – is what matters, just as what matters in the telling of an illness narrative is that it conveys 'effectively' a semblance of a world in which the writer bears his or her pain.

Only when artistic skill and the artist's illness history (the person's biography) are brought together does the autopathography emerge, or the work of illness come into being. By imagining the world transformed there arises the possibility of re-envisioning its ordinary properties. This is not a static state but a tension or movement between the two spheres, something that is apprehended – or one might better say, entertained – through aesthetic sensibilities. In works of art this tension is not exterior but an essential aspect of their interior construction, and facilitated in autobiography and painting through exemplifications of the artist's life.

A clear example (perhaps in its clarity making it untypical) is provided by one of Martha Hall's artist's books, titled 'One Week from Today'. It is described in the catalogue to the exhibition, Holding In, Holding On as a 'Three part portfolio covered with hand-made Cave Paper enclosing loose sheets of the artist's hand-made paper. Hand-made paper with collage, printing (colograph and photo transfer) and chine colle. Handwritten with brown colored pencils.' (Hall, 2003). On one page a transfer of Martha Hall's face can be discerned against the background, with red pencil crosses at her chin and at the corner of her right eye. A red line joins the two crosses. The accompanying verse (written on the book pages) opens with the words:

> 'I must have an X-ray on Monday,
> One week from today.
>
> They will search for cancer in the bone behind my eye.'

and then moves to another sphere:

> 'Let there be another answer –
> Wintergreen, solvents,
> Printer's ink.
>
> I have stood this week in the sun,
> Pulling color from the water
> Onto my pages.'

The poem continues with examples of Hall's transformation of the world:

> 'I have heard the stories
> Of the blacksmith with pearls,
>
> And seen the grace and intensity of the juggler.
>
> I have seen the coiled ropes in the
> Wet woods –
> Wondered if made by artist or fisherman.'

And then returns to the mundane via the lines:

> 'I have held a salted fish in my hands,
> Its scales pearlescent inspiration.'

Then concludes in the place at which we found her:

> 'This week I am an artist.
> Next week is one week from today.'

To read this book is therefore to be told about Hall's life through the poem and also to know it through handling the book with its hand-made pages.

The art and the illness experience are co-extensive in the screen that she creates to convey her situation.

That a poor writer might also create a moving account, or that many ill people do not have the skills to create artworks in this genre is not the issue. Nor does it matter if the author/artist makes the work as part of a political project, in the course of which the evocation of illness is such as to inspire others to feel themselves co-sufferers. What is crucial for seeing a work as 'autopathography' is the sense of a duality in the artist/sufferer. The compassion felt on this occasion is to be distinguished from that felt when seeing, *in vivo*, an unfortunate or a person in suffering. Then the appropriate response is immediate action so as to relieve distress, grounded in being directly touched by that suffering. In the case of reading or viewing works of illness, the response is neither ameliorating action to change the (mundane) world, nor is it an aesthetic appreciation of the way that suffering has been rendered in the world of art. Both of these responses presume a separation of the spheres that works of illness attempt to conjoin in the fabrication of the text, or in the arrangement of light and shapes. To understand the response to such works we need to see that what they do is to transform suffering and re-present it in forms made accessible through the responses and acts of the afflicted persons. It is not horror as such that is looked in the face in these depictions but its configuration in the actions of the authors and artists concerned. It is their 'way of looking' (at illness) that is mediated by the story or the picture, and which is made available to the reader and viewer.

In artistic renderings, made by a third party, the spectator might be said to 'sympathise with the painter', who has established an asymmetrical relationship with the afflicted person. One outcome of this asymmetry is that the afflicted person is identified with his or her suffering, but is not seen to rise above it. In consequence, the objection is raised by activists about exhibitions of photographs of people as victims of this or that disease. The political response to this is to create a system of places (an epidemiology) distinct from the individuals who occupy them (Boltanski, 1999: 120, Patton, 1995). These actions are integral within a world of jurisdictions where rights prevail, and in which aesthetic values (tastes, sensibilities) are seen as irrelevant, or worse still, contribute to the stigmatisation of afflicted individuals and their group.

However, in the case of 'autopathographies' and self-portraits, the asymmetry between artist and subject is brokered in a different way, most obviously in the fact that the artist and the sufferer are the same person. Rather than depending primarily upon distinctions in a world of discourse, these works are primarily self-presentations where the artist displays his or her condition through exemplifying it. The self-referential quality of these works detaches (but does not remove) them from being subject to the criteria of the political sphere. While every work of art is self-announcing – entire to itself – works of illness, dealing as they do with horror as well as compassion, engage the reader in a reversible asymmetry expressed by the author/sufferer, or artist/sufferer figured in the work concerned. We do not see just suffering but rather individuals 'rising in their suffering' (Frank, 1998:340). This duality finds its correspondence in the tension created in the reader/observer; the idea of how the world 'might or could be' calls out a response in his or her orientation to the world. Another way of putting this is to say that the problematisation of illness envisaged by the artist or author touches the viewer, not by bringing her to tears (necessarily), but by *re-locating her* in relation to a vulnerability that is sought out in her by the work. As Boltanski says:

> ...by painting the unfortunate's suffering, by revealing its horror and thereby revealing its truth, he confers on this suffering the only form of dignity to which it can lay claim and which it gets from its attachment to the world of the already painted, of what has already been revealed within an aesthetic register. ... the presentation of the unfortunate in his horrific aspect is the only one which makes possible the communication of that unpresentable horror which overcomes the spectator and which is none other than the horror residing within him and which defines his condition (Boltanski, 1999: 116).

On this basis we can see that the duality that a third party discerns in the artist/author is fundamental to the apprehension of the story, painting or photograph *as a particular kind of work*. This apprehension of duality is also key to its emergence as a corresponding state in the viewer or reader. Works of illness do not so much provide an affirmation of being itself (as in being touched in the flesh) but more an affirmation of a *way* of being, something premised upon an idea of suffering that provokes an ethical as well as an aesthetic response.

The Gift of Presence

All works *about* illness are not works *of* illness. This is sometimes the judgement on photographs of the sick made by others, and can be said of accounts that, even when written by ex-patients, are couched in a style that objectifies their topic. To evoke that sublimity central to the work being 'touching' requires that they do something different from pictures or accounts that primarily denote and specify. In a nutshell, what works of illness have to do is to *re-present* for a third party that experience to which the sufferer was initially prey, but in the execution of the work, to show herself as witness. This end is achieved when the third party is brought together with the author/artist in relation to the work, when sympathy *for* the afflicted is surpassed by sympathy *with* them for what has been faced and (possibly, but not necessarily) overcome.

This way of signifying is different from denoting or designating, the primary mode of scientific endeavour, which Latour (1988, 1998) says is the work of 'immutable mobiles'. The emergence of science as a regime of representation involved the re-inscription of features on different media, so that what eventually came to be seen as measures or indices defined different classes of objects that could be manipulated at a distance. The holding constant of certain key indices, as measures, across different media is what constitutes immutability; the potential for applying these measures across temporal and spatial contexts is what makes them mobile. This regime displaced a medieval one that operated, in Europe, in the realm of Christian religious painting. And it is in works of religion that we find strong parallels with works of illness.

Latour argues that the aim – the rationale – of religious paintings is not to depict accurately stories from the Bible as if to prove scientifically that such and such an event occurred. It is rather to bring into the presence of the viewer – as third party – the experience of people depicted – apostles and saints – in relation to Jesus. The aim of these works is therefore not depiction for accuracy's sake, but to show forth, expressively, 'our' relationship to God. It is to make a 'gift of presence' to the viewer where that refers to a re-presentation made possible by a contemplation of the scene shown.

> In person making what counts above all, what requires the utmost sacrifice, is the designation, here and now, of the person at hand, being presented with the gift of presence. But there is no way to produce this effect by directing attention away from the scene. On the contrary, the only way is to *redirect* attention by pointing, through the cracks in the discourse, to the character in the flesh listening to the story or watching the scene. (Latour, 1998: 429, emphasis in original).

This redirection of attention is important, because it indicates the functional difference between signifiers that denote objects, pointing away into a world of other places and other times, and signifiers that are infra-referential with regard to the picture being viewed (or the story being heard). It is through the latter kind that the viewer is invited to reconstruct the route of the signifiers (cf. the 'route of the heart') in order to complete the arc that was begun by the artist. In that sense, religious pictures were (prior to the emergence of scientific representation) mutable in the sense that they re-presented their message anew with each viewing, opening up the potential (though not the certainty) of the viewer receiving 'the gift of life anew' (Latour, 1998). The message then is about *the viewers/readers currently engaging the work*, and what these individuals might do *now*. For Latour, the key to this infra- or self-reference is the use of signifiers that are extra-discursive, in the sense that what he calls 'the arrows' are pointing 'through the cracks, discrepancies, visual puzzles, absurdities of the scene' so as to locate again the third party in relation to God (1998: 431). The idea of being *located again* carries the important point that, like affirmations of love, these messages are not exhausted – are not exhaustible – in the telling.

To illustrate this idea we can look again at the photograph '*I Framed my Breast for Posterity*', (see Figure 2). Spence selected this photograph as being exemplary of the form that 'a photography for the sick' might take (Dennett, 2001). Spence is naked from the waist up, except for a string of wooden beads. On the underside of her left breast is a bandage. The beads and bandage mark (colonize) her body and connect this photograph to a pair of photographs titled 'Colonization' that she and Dennett had made earlier that year, before her diagnosis of breast cancer (Spence, 1988). To the left of her head is a black and white poster of a group of British mineworkers, who were engaged in collective action at the time. Below the poster is a fireplace, with a fire burning in the grate. On the mantelpiece are an alarm clock, a tin mug, and a greeting card. To the right of Spence and partially covering the wall is a brown-coloured fabric screen, printed with large, bright red flowers, used to obscure a window from appearing in the picture.

This is a carefully composed photograph, essentially a tableau, in the sense that it is posed, makes use of props and has been carefully lit from below (Dennett, p.c.). This enhances its look – its shock. The narrative the Spence provides is essential to understanding this photograph. And yet the picture is not reducible to a narrative in that the pictorial arrangement of signifiers works to make this picture self-announcing. The photograph's effect comes from disrupting conventions in order to make signs work in a way that proposes authorship ('there is a message here'). This also means there is a message *here*, *now*, in the sense of Lyotard's (1984) gloss on the shock of the 'sublime' in modern art. Inviting the viewer to look at her, Spence (as figured) looks back so that the viewer is brought before the picture: both representation and viewer are made present to each other.

While Spence's deliberate presentation of herself bare breasted against the ordinariness of the background is unexpected (disruptive), it is the use of the picture frame that directs the viewer's attention to the 'sick' breast with its bandage. Not only is this breast being made visible: its appearance is made ambiguous by it being 'pictured within the picture'. At a mundane level it is Spence herself who is pictured. But at an imaginary level the picture frame that encloses her breast at the same time de-realizes it. This serves to displace it from the everyday and makes it into a double signifier that exists in mundane and imaginary worlds at once. As sufferer and artist, Spence is both figure and person, the maker and the made. It is in the relationship between these aspects that the authenticity of the work is to be sought and tried. The test of this cannot be against information in the everyday world of facts and politics because the picture (and the autobiographical text) attains its truth via a different route. It is similar to the 'route of the heart', as Boltanski calls it, as it refers to a test of *witness*, not one of artistic skill or empirical analysis.

But this relocation is not redemptive, certainly not in the religious sense of the word. While the horrors of illness are not denoted, they are potentiated in the title of Spence's picture that alludes to what is to happen to her. However, the 'arrows' (to use Latour's word) draw attention to Spence's illness experience by taking aside the gaze, by the act of picturing within the picture. The use of re-organised visual symbols can also be considered to act as 'discursive safety harnesses' that allow viewers to enter into the pit of fear she shows them and to contemplate what it means for any woman to face the prospect of breast removal. There is no guarantee here that all viewers will see the same things because the visual engagement with the picture and the cultural frames surrounding breast cancer will vary with different viewers, especially women with breast cancer. However, for each viewer, Spence's photograph is an invitation to contemplate her situation, by thinking about it, or by talking about it between themselves. This is a matter of sharing, of collective meaning, of discourse. But no matter how much we talk about it we do not exhaust this photograph of its meaning. The picture does not dissolve in discourse nor, as we find out more about the reasons for its construction, do we want it to. As with other works, both visual and textual, it has the potential, with each engagement, to re-locate the viewer in relation to its subject, facing serious illness.

This significant property of paintings is not a once and for all announcement but an indication that meaning is to be *sought* on the canvas. The 'cracks in the discourse' are not limited to disruptions to visual symbols but become foregrounded in the act of looking and searching that the painting demands. Whereas to denote is to point to an entity, be it concrete or abstract, to exemplify is to indicate which property or feature amongst those on display is the appropriate referent (Goodman, 1978). In that sense exemplification is fecund because 'every property of an example is a *prima facie* candidate for securing the referent.' (Silvers, 1978: 41). Having said that, the organization of a painting is such as to restrict or otherwise condition that candidature in order to express its meaning. One of the key skills in picturing or describing illness experience is to deploy signs and features in a way that both announces the work, and enables the viewer to reconstruct its message.

What of autobiographical stories of illness? These are not pictures yet the work that authors have to do is the same with respect to making its reading an occasion, a story that has significance for the reader who is prepared to listen. Where self-portraits show the relationship of artist to illness in the simultaneous deployment of signs, the autobiographical account uses narrative means to indicate this relationship, while yet calling attention to the way that the reader should 'follow the route' of the story. 'Autopathographies' are not 'just stories', if only because they must show again the feature that inspired the telling. The first person account must display, in some sense, the author's pain, and thereby induce the reader to appreciate the world of his or her suffering. And to extend this point, the third person commentary must, in similar vein, preserve and show again those features of the sufferer's story that struck them when they first heard it.

In a discussion of medical ethics and doctoring, Carson (1995) picks out an extract from Arthur Frank's (1991) book *At the Will of the Body*. Frank described hearing about his diagnosis of cancer in a medical consultation:

> By then I felt less terrorized by the idea of cancer than validated by a recognition that I was seriously ill… Even though my worst fears were realized in what he said, the physician showed, *just by the way he looked at me and a couple of phrases he used*, that he shared in the seriousness of my situation. The vitality of his support was as personal as it was professional' (Frank, *At the Will of the Body*, quoted by Carson, 1995: 123. emphasis added.)

Carson argues that the words, 'just by the way he looked at me and a couple of phrases he used' are signs of recognition given to Frank by his doctor. That is, they are indicative of an act of imagination on the part of the doctor, showing that he has understood his patient's situation. This recognition completes the arc of understanding that Frank, as witness, uses to show us, as readers, what he was going through. What is significant here (what we might call the *mediation*) is the report of the doctor's way of looking and the unspecified phrases he used. These two, quite specific descriptions appear as features that situate the moment in a particular way. They set out a *co-incidence* that tells of the doctor's re-positioning in relation to Arthur Frank's plight. In being reported, the descriptions form a break in the flow of the story, insofar as they refer to the 'way of showing' by which Frank felt himself acknowledged by the doctor. This break – a crack in the discourse – is made significant by showing to the reader the moment when Arthur Frank's suffering was re-configured in the act of being witnessed by another (his doctor). This re-configuration is not something that can be communicated adequately by being merely denoted. Instead, to be shown forth, it must be brought into the presence of the reader, alluding to Frank's situation in the eyes of his physician. In a sense, the reader needs to be *shown* certain essential features of this moment that place it as an act of witnessing.

Witnessing at Second Hand: research as showing

We have seen that works of illness must show the relationship of sufferer to illness as witness, and they do this through making cracks in the discourse, as an ascetic and aesthetic endeavour. It would be wrong, however, to think that this way of showing is restricted only to autobiographic works. There are published reports that attempt this through description of the person's suffering at the time. Equally important, the author *as witness* of the event described must be distinguished from, and then brought into relation to the author *as researcher* reporting the study.

In their account of a doctor's interview with a woman patient from Haiti, Katz and Shotter (1996) attempt to show the potential of what they call a 'social poetics' for understanding a person's inner world of pain. They pay special attention to both the medical discourse and to what they refer to as the 'local talk' between the doctor and patient. This allows an examination of the significance of shifts in the patient's dialogue with the doctor, and thus the fleeting moments that capture the emergence of the patient's own voice. Katz designates her presence at the consultation in terms of a distinct role as 'cultural go-between'. In this role, she heard the woman say, in a brief response to the doctor's question, "It's not like that back home. It's hard to work there [in the nursing home in the US]. I'm working too hard". From this position Katz reports:

> As she said it, there was a marked shift in the intensity of her speech, a slowing down, a process punctuated by shifts in her posture…. a looking down to her left and a sinking-in-on-herself…. a sense of despair darkened her story. Her saying "It's not like it is back home" seemed

> suddenly, at that moment, to come from 'somewhere else'. I was
> occupied by what was not said but gestured. Something gave color and
> life to the stark symptoms picture, something from her life, her culture.
> (Katz and Shotter, 1996: 921).

Katz-as-researcher goes on to say that she was struck by this brief occurrence, wonders why it moved her so powerfully and was guided by its underlying significance in her analysis of the whole consultation. She examines this in terms of the way the words "It's not like that back home" present a gap in the flow of the discourse, a discontinuity communicated in terms of a 'deep sadness and withdrawal, shown in her whole expression of it, in her voicing, in her gesturing of it.' (Katz and Shotter, 1996: 922). What these authors go on to argue is that these 'arresting moments' in medical dialogue are both indicators of significant changes in voice and also opportunities for increased understanding of the patient's lifeworld.

What is interesting about this example is that it presents the significance of the exchange in terms of Katz's own reaction to the moment. It is not so much the words that are said – although they are important – but also the manner in which they were spoken, a manner that is inseparable from Katz's apprehension of it. This was not mere gesture but a deep sadness that, she says, 'hung in the air and was palpable between us, yet ignored.' (1996: 922). What the recognition of this moment meant was that the woman could be asked to speak from that personal or local position, to give voice to concerns that were excluded by the requirement that she speak within the framework of medical discourse.

This example is pertinent here because it poses the question of what the recognition of this discontinuity means for understanding the voice of the ill person. Just as with the break in the discourse described by Arthur Frank, here we have a discontinuity that is preserved in the account in order to locate a qualitative shift in understanding. At one level this is a movement away from silence towards an explication of the ill person's world. Where previously the sufferer could not speak, now she is able to do so. (Katz and Shotter go on to describe how the Hiatian woman could articulate her lifeworld, once signalled that her own voice would be heard). However, at another level, there remains an unarticulated aspect of both sufferers' positions, which is the recognition of the 'gap in signification' itself. And this is important, because the preservation of the sense of that moment must be conveyed (as it is in both excerpts quoted above) in order that readers can be brought into the presence of the same conditions that provoked this discontinuity.

What this example shows is the duality displayed within the picture or autobiography being created, as it were, in the course of a third party report of another's pain. While not a work of art, Katz and Shotter's report uses its poetic stance to *re-present* the moment in which the woman's pain appeared. We need to go one step further to establish that the 'cracks in the discourse' that we see 'all at once' on a canvas, or set out in narrative form in a book, can be created between people using different media. The intention is to demonstrate that the aesthetic portrayal of witnessing extends, potentially, to contexts beyond the painted canvas and the autobiographical account of illness.

The emotion that this woman showed was a 'gesture' toward a world in which, though never explicated, was nevertheless shown to be significant. This significance was perceived because her emotion was not only being represented – denoted – but because it was being shown forth in the way she spoke. This might be called the 'tone of voice', were it not that tone is a property of the speaking voice that, though it changes, is a constant aspect of speech that properly belongs to it. By comparison, what Barthes called the 'grain of the voice' is a summary term for the way that the woman expressed her situation. The 'grain of the voice' is not an inherent property but is metaphorically possessed by it, referring to features of the person's illness world. (For Barthes this 'grain' might be, 'the body in the voice as it sings, the hand as it writes, the limb as it performs' (1977: 188). We are dealing here with a voice that communicates not merely by being turned on, having been presumptively silenced. Instead, the voice of the woman made its appearance with the exemplification of her world. This might be spoken, written, or painted – or just indicated by means of bodily posture. In every case, the manner of its appearance is what is indicative of the moment – the space-time it creates – and of the semantic potential with which it invites others to engage.

The expression of emotion in this context invites a response that is participatory on the part of the clinician or researcher (as third party), a response that enters into the moment or the space that this display makes possible. This response might not be forthcoming, either because the other does not wish to make it, or simply because the display is not recognised by him/her as exemplary of a world. However, where it is so recognised, this is more of an endorsement of an opportunity to let the person tell their story or to elaborate that display into a local discourse. What matters (as was shown in Carson's gloss on Arthur Frank's account of his meeting with his doctor) is that the speaking and the listening together expand upon the space that is created in the recognition of the gesture as exemplary. In her work on narrative medicine Rita Charon describes how, as a doctor, she invites this space with the words to her patients, 'I will be your doctor, and so I must learn a great deal about your body and your health and your life. Please tell me what you think I should know about your situation' (Charon, 2009). As an example, she tells of sitting with a woman with muscular dystrophy, as close as possible, thigh to thigh, in order to try to inhabit her climate of panicky despair and not to leave her alone in it. In this example, the participatory act is anticipatory and invitational, not just of a mood, but of an occasion in which the patient might lay down her story alongside those told by the doctor (Radley, Mayberry and Pearce, 2008).

A key part of telling about these occasions is that the status of the gesture – the break in the discourse – is not explicable in terms of the patient alone. The recognition of the gesture is not contained in the illness narrative, but is 'made into' something by the third party who witnesses it, or even encourages it. And this is achieved through descriptions that make reference to the situation in which the stories were told – not just to gestures, but to the others present, to the setting and to other forms of representation apart from talk that either exemplify or denote aspects of the person's world as it appeared to the investigator. The sufferer's world makes its appearance in a setting that it partly creates. This can only happen because the setting is transformed when the researcher apprehends what the person's gesture exemplifies. The apprehension of the gesture as making a critical moment (as infra-reflexive) is another way of saying that the occasion is made by its appearance. Then the researcher says that new possibilities for telling arose in the consultation, or that aspects of the interview situation became explicable or could be used to throw light on what the patient had but barely talked about. Changes in posture or facial expression, or in the doctor's tone of voice, are features that become salient when taken up in the occasions they help to figure.

Therefore, to display one's suffering anew (and every meeting with another is a new context) is to display references that have not been established prior to that encounter. The mediation that will be employed and the properties that might be cross-referred do not lie inside the person who suffers, but are taken up in the context (the relationship, the setting) in which the meeting takes place. It is not certain what these will be, or which new ones will arise. One thing that is certain is that the fabrication of this as an occasion – something that takes place in a space of its own making – means that potentially anything in the situation can be made to signify or can afterwards appear so. Then the researcher might remember the room in which they met the person – or their clothes, or the weather, or a number of features that now signify in the telling of the person's story. Both parties are opened up to the surroundings in which their exchange takes place – not as a physical context, but in terms of those features that might 'best' exemplify the world that the patient shows forth. This space is an opening into the idea or the feeling in terms of which suffering is exemplified. The moment is a fragment, a figuration, of a world of illness. In the case of the Haitian woman patient, Katz (as cultural go-between) says, 'I found myself wondering again about what was not said, but hung, arrested, in the space between us, creating a silence that was anything but silent: 'What is her suffering about?' (Katz and Shotter, 1996: 922)

If we think of this as being, at the time, an anticipatory posture of the 'researcher when present' (rather than an articulated question made subsequently in a report) then there is an openness to finding out which features in the situation are crucial to understanding the suffering being shown. Which cracks in the discourse are to be followed? Acknowledging that something important is being portrayed here sets in train an act of looking that seeks across all of the terrain that agonistic space then offers. (One looks at the person's face, at their posture, listens to what they say, and perhaps hears (without listening!) the ticking of the clock in the silence created when the person does not speak. The communication of suffering, as discussed here, is akin to a replete symbol, (of which paintings are a good example), in which every mark, line or colour tone has semantic potential. As Goodman says, 'the search for accurate adjustment between symbol and symbolized calls for maximal sensitivity, and is unending' (1968: 236). That is why presentational displays offer not a specification but a metaphorical representation that is multiplied, disrupted and cross-referenced by the mediation. The work of exemplification in reporting serious illness is to show 'how suffering might be', displayed in context features that allude, for example, to its colour (blue), its elevation (depressed), its posture (slumped) and its rhythm (dragging).

This idea about portrayal as being different to denotation raises the point that there are limits to the visual: the figurative portrayal of an illness world cannot be isolated on the canvas or print because it is not there to be seen. We should have respect not for 'the image itself' but for its mode of presentation, because 'there is *nothing to see* when we do a freeze-frame of scientific and religious practice and focus on the visual' (Latour, 1998:421, emphasis in original). There is 'nothing to see' in the sense that the meaning of the work can be designated in, and therefore located on particular parts of the picture. This is equally true of stories of suffering, where discourse is the medium for the portrayal of 'suffering-as-borne'. In each case – picture and narrative – any search for meaning in the formal properties of the medium fails to embrace the aesthetic (and ethical) dimension at the root of its comprehension (Frank, 2000b). The portrayal of 'persons' rather than 'objects' involves a re-designation of the viewer as someone receiving the message or the picture anew. This fashioning of the other's illness world 'within' the observer constitutes the re-figuration of him/her with respect to the mundane world of pain and suffering. This re-figuring is coterminous with a sense of having received the message of the work, and shows that signification, in this case, is not to do with communicating meaning about objects, but is all about the instantiation of persons.

Looking and Listening Out

There is no way that pictures and stories can guarantee an effect, or deliver a particular message to each and every reader or viewer. There will always be differences in the readiness of people to engage with any work, let alone one that invites them into a world of horror or suffering. We have already touched on the fact that feelings of pity and compassion might be amplified or muted by the social identity of the sufferer or needy person. At this point I want to take up the readiness of some people to engage with works of illness, and how that readiness might translate into them following not just 'the route of the heart' but 'the route of the work'. Among the most eligible individuals will be those who also suffer from the particular disease portrayed in the story, or those who have been touched by serious illness or those close to them. Artworks have become rallying points for people with AIDS and for women with breast cancer, as any search of the Internet will reveal. However, merely to say which groups of viewers or readers are likely to engage with works like this is not the point. Rather, by examining the situation of those most ready for this can we say more about how stories and pictures do their work. The presumption is that people with serious illness already have their lives disrupted to some degree, their biographic constituents shaken to the point of needing re-assembly.

The cultural theorist Jackie Stacey provides a fascinating illustration of readiness in her book *Teratologies* (Stacey, 1997). Most of her book is taken up with an account of the way that cancer is researched and represented, as well as the way in which it is treated within the regime of Western medicine. As well as this, she tells a story about her own experience of cancer, her diagnosis, treatment and recovery. Jackie Stacey was diagnosed as having an endodermal sinus tumour, a highly malignant tumour of the egg cell. Following a course of chemotherapy, she recuperated with a friend by renting a cottage on the Greek island of Crete. As a result of the chemotherapy she had lost her eyebrows, eyelashes, and hair so that in consequence, as she put it, 'certainly no one looked like me.' That is, until one day in the town nearby she saw coming towards her a young woman who also had that 'uncannily naked look'. She reports that, 'She looked completely familiar and yet totally unfamiliar at the same time. Did I do a double-take, or do I just imagine I did? How obvious was the shock in my expression? (Stacey, 1997: 18)

Stacey and the woman (who had been treated for the same rare form of cancer, a most unlikely coincidence) did not speak but passed by each other, so that she returned home with a yearning, the 'longing for the might-have-been of recognition'. Later on she introduced herself to this woman; they compared their illness experiences, so similar in many details that when Stacey returned to her apartment she says, 'I wept with relief'.

Stacey reflects on this extraordinary meeting by saying:

> For me, this encounter is the story of my re-entry into the social world after weeks of claustrophobic internality in my physical body.... The presence of another (similar but not the same, like me but not like me) enabled me to make a crucial transition out of the frozen shock of the treatment and into the world of narrative exchange. Her story made sense of mine. And my story gained substance as she listened. (Stacey, 1997: 20)

What is it that Stacey recognised *with relief*? We can conjecture that it was herself-as-ill in the other woman, an-other whose existence produces the conditions for dialogue, a space in which to speak and also to listen. So while the dialogue enabled comparisons to be made, this discursive space was first made possible by recognition, in which the *similar (but not the same)* was mapped onto itself in a mimetic act. Mimesis here is akin to a co-incidence, in the sense that certain aspects of the mediation were made salient, and potentiated the naming (through dialogue) of experiences both women had undergone. We might further conjecture that the 'cracks' that had appeared in Stacey's life as a result of cancer, involving her body and her social appearance, resonated with those offered by the appearance of this other woman. In an extraordinary meeting, it might be said – not merely literally, but in the sense offered by Lacan (1979) – that not only did both women (as perceivers) look, but that both women (*as perceived*) looked back.

In discussing the example in this way I have moved through the story so to speak, relying upon Stacey's description to try to grasp what might be involved in recognition, not just of another real person, but of a figured individual. Stacey's story is relevant to any reader – and particularly to those people who might have cancer – for its message of the occurrence of something 'too fictional to ever hope for, yet too coincidental to belong in good fiction'. (1997: 19). It is made relevant by the careful construction of descriptive passages – what Riessman (1990) called those 'touching non-narrative passages' – that enable an empathic appreciation of what we are being told. In the case of works of illness, the disruptions and cracks, alluding to the artist/writer's experience in the world shared by viewers and readers, will resonate differently with individuals who look out from variously different positions of need.

Somewhere between the meeting in real life and the fabricated picture lies the documentary photograph. Looking at one such photograph of Jo Spence receiving a mammography, Susan Bell wrote that, 'The photograph of her huge squeezed breast compels viewers, *especially women*, to respond in a visceral way to the image by putting themselves into the picture and one of their own breasts into the space occupied by Spence's breast' (Bell, 2002: 23-24, emphasis added). This putting of one breast in place of another, one which is similar (but not the same), shows again the mimetic act in which discursive space is ruptured (is 'cracked') if only temporarily to enable dialogue to take place. The 'visceral' response to which Bell draws attention is nothing less than the challenge to *name* what this 'becoming similar to' represents. Whatever it is, the recognition of a common fate, a shared experience, can be a validating and empowering experience that works of illness make possible.

However, the meeting that Jackie Stacey describes *in* the story is not a work of illness. To move to a genetic analysis of that meeting is to trace out 'the route of the heart', in which the mutual sympathetic response is one of co-presence, made corporeal in the tears of relief that Stacey sheds, for herself, for the other woman, and for their shared situation. But works of illness do not evoke sympathy in the form associated with a face-to-face meeting with a suffering person. Works of art set out an idea, create their meaning through achieving an ascetic distance between the artist and the fabricated screen, of paint, of words. In the case of pictures and stories, this screen, with all its self-announcing 'arrows', figures the artist/author in a way that presents them as witness *of something*. That something is the semblance of an idea concerning illness, horror or suffering, so that to know it (even if one cannot name it) is to see as the artist/author. This grasping of the act of witness can only follow from the viewer/reader *'tracing the route of the work'*, which is to move back and forth across the various disruptions, cracks, and diversions that are offered in small descriptive passages, juxtapositions of text and photograph, unexpected pictorial arrangements or textures of light and shade.

Works of illness, offered as agonistic portrayals, are not aimed primarily at establishing a sympathetic response to the artist or author concerned. What is offered in these works is a different, and potentially new way of looking and knowing the world. Dealing in acts of witness and in semblances rather than in specifications, they offer the opportunity for readers and viewers to realise their world differently, whether as fellow sufferers or not. In both cases, those individuals become co-witnesses, and by internalising the 'route of the work', can take it again and again into their own everyday experience. This for example, is true in the case of photographs where Jo Spence places herself in the picture, her breasts exposed, displaying the marks of her biopsy. She invites a shock of recognition from fellow sufferers as well as an engagement and self-reflection by those who have not (yet) been diagnosed with breast cancer (Bell, 2002, 2006). This invitation is repeated for women with breast cancer in every exhibition attended and in every book opened in the years since these photographs were made. This makes possible, at one moment, the visibility of breast cancer as the common situation (the 'likeness') of women who are similarly afflicted.

What do works of illness do, when treated agonistically, if they do not trade in sympathy? Some would say that they are empowering, or person making, or provide the gift of presence. They do these things but also, by creating a semblance of how things are, they lift the viewer/reader's eyes to the landscape of illness, so that one can sense, if not see it for what it is. Ascetic distance is not merely some artistic device, nor just a redemptive strategy but the essence of what we termed earlier on, the problematisation of illness as an act of freedom. Although artworks recruit our elusory powers for their effect, their aim is ultimately to dis-illusion us about the world. Virginia Woolf unmasked the elevation of sympathy in saying:

> There is, let us confess it, (and illness is a great confessional) a childish outspokenness in illness: things are said, truths blurted out, which the cautious respectability of health conceals. About sympathy for example; we can do without it. That illusion of the world so shaped that it echoes every groan, of human beings so tied together by common needs and fears that a twitch at one wrist jerks another, where however strange your experience other people have had it too, where however far you travel in your own mind someone has been there before you – is all an illusion. …. Human beings do not go hand in hand the whole stretch of the way. There is a virgin forest, tangled, pathless, in each; a snowfield where even the print of birds' feet is unknown. Here we go alone, and

like it better so. Always to have sympathy, always to be accompanied, always to be understood, would be intolerable. But in health the genial pretence must be kept up and the effort renewed ... In illness this make-believe ceases. (1994: 320-321)

This idea is consistent with the view that stories and pictures about illness do not convey answers that shore up fragile selves, or indeed that such works are about the 'self' of author or reader, artist or viewer. Tracing meaning back inside – to the emotional drive of the artist or the emotional response of the viewer – simply misses the point that these works are about the fabrication of worlds, the transmutation of the real and the imaginary. Rather like the religious paintings considered by Latour, they offer the 'gift of presence' by inviting viewers/readers to join in witness, so that what they attain, in turn, is the ascetic distance on which a figured world depends. Put simply, it is the gift of being able to bear witness to one's own and other people's illness situation.

In the light of these comments, it is instructive to think of works of illness as being gifts which, when they cross boundaries, abolish the boundary altogether. By comparison, commodities – or inscriptions that are denotatively derived – cross lines without changing their nature (they are immutable) or else they establish a boundary where there was none before (Hyde, 1999: 61). Sociological explanations of narratives, and analyses of the formal properties of visual representations are examples of the latter kind of inscription; their immutability is why they are of limited aesthetic and ethical worth to individuals who are seriously ill. In the Maussian sense, perhaps there is a social obligation involved in the receiving of such a gift, which is to pass it on. What to pass on? One's own story perhaps, or to listen more attentively to the stories of others? To engage with fellow sufferers in acts of witness whose aim is to raise public consciousness about disease, even though this means a different way of using such works, as in activist programmes? This would square with Mauss's description of communal gift giving as not being the circulation of the same object (the same story need not be re-told). And we cannot, for obvious reasons, return a gift to the artist or the author.

If we examine this idea of 'the gift' a little more closely, it bears out some of the things that have been said so far about the way that artworks might function in the creation of a sympathetic body of witnesses. The well-known analysis that Mauss (1966) makes of Maori gift exchange has at its centre the idea that objects carry the spirit of *hau*, a spirit that is made manifest in traditional community exchanges. It operates as follows. Person B receives something (without obligation) from Person A. Person B then makes a similar kind of gift (though not of the same object) to Person C. At some later time Person B receives a gift from Person C, which s/he cannot retain lest s/he fall ill or even die. This object carries the *hau* (spirit) that in its returning trajectory must not be impeded but fostered by B, who must give something back to Person A. While a gift is free of payment it is not free of obligation – far from it. In his Malinowski Memorial Lecture, Parry made the important point that 'the ideology of a disinterested gift emerges in parallel with an ideology of a purely interested exchange' (Parry, 1986: 458), which is to say, in this context, that ideas about art as gift need to be seen in the context of modern day consumerism. What consumerism separates is person from thing (or work), spirit from body, which is precisely what is retained in a gift that one person makes for another. We might better think of the recipient of such a gift as being someone who, to gloss Mauss's discussion of the Germanic tribes, is constrained to make a return 'since he has handed over as pledge an object which is imbued with his own personality, and which therefore puts him, quite literally in the hands of his creditor. By redeeming it he redeems himself.' (Parry, 1986: 457).

Works of illness – insofar as they are pictures or stories about one's illness – have a self-referential potential that restores the commonality of object and person. The story that is told or the picture that is shown is the ground on which is established the duality of the person as both artist and sufferer, perceived together as witness. What is received, as in Martha Hall's experience recounted in the story of the man with the tattoo of Curious George, is both insight and obligation, which in her case was the need to 'make art' about her illness and to pass this on. The obligation was felt in the duality that the man's story potentiated in her. By making her artists' books, she made available works in which others could locate their own illness experience, and related to which all who can see attest to what they have seen. In recounting her story of Curious George she also made some return of the gift. As Arthur Frank has put it, '*in order to be generous, first be grateful*' (2004: 142). What is owed returns not to the person as a separate individual, but to the work as product of witness. We have here, in parallel with the circulating gift, the basis of a community body established in the sequential (mimetic) placing of oneself as listener, viewer, sufferer and maker of art (or teller of stories).

We cannot assume, however, that a reader or viewer knows how or when to pass on what they have received in reading a story or in viewing a picture. The ascetic distance established by laying on paint, composing a photograph, or writing a book is less easily achieved by those who are neither artists nor writers. There remains an openness here that is inevitable, and for that reason potentially productive. For example, after reading a description of listening to the accounts of MS sufferers, the sociologist Elizabeth Chaplin wrote, 'When I read that text, I begin to rethink my life as a woman, as a sociologist and even as a potential sufferer from a disease which is difficult to diagnose. I want to know more because Wynne's way of writing makes what she says seem relevant for my future life.' (1994: 269). And for that to happen we see why the work must also relate in some way to the world of the viewer and reader. It is through the joint participation in the presentational form of witnessing that the viewer/reader enters into the imaginative act that is the aesthetic projection. By itself this guarantees little, if only because to produce its effects the aesthetic mode must refract – must pass through – everyday (ideological) concerns over which it comes to have figurative control. This is another way of saying that the aesthetic is not ethereal but takes up the mundane world in which people dwell jointly, for example as women, or as sociologists.

Finally, like all gifts, works of illness are not exhausted through re-presentation. The individuals who make them have established, in their turn, a position of witness that opens up further possibilities, both in terms of creating other works and also in making choices in life. In the case of people with serious disease, their future life is one that involves recovery, some kind of remission or even a decline leading to death. In each of these cases the person making the work has different opportunities to use their stories or pictures as they will. This involves both the continued display of the works for others, through publishing, workshops or exhibitions, and the use of these works in the mundane world of their own illness, as a way of keeping alive. The potential for works of illness to have a redemptive function, as they constitute a figurative affirmation of health, is the topic to which I now turn.

Chapter 4

Remedy and Redemption

Stories and pictures about illness secure their significance in a number of locations, or with reference to several points in time. This might be the result of their having roots in both the imaginary and the mundane. Also, these stories and pictures extend their messages – of whatever kind – to other people and, inevitably, to the authors/artists themselves. To the degree that these messages are positive, there is the implication that works of illness are more than symptomatic of illness; they are somehow indexical of 'recovery and return', a 'symptom of not dying' (Stacey, 1997: 241). This implies that they do not merely reflect recovery, but are partly constitutive of it. Towards the end of her book Jackie Stacey wonders if writing her cultural account of cancer – of cancer in general – is a defence against her own mortality. She even wonders whether she hesitates to finish the book, because in writing it she is somehow protected from death. But there is also the possibility that, by embedding what happened to her in the context of public explanations of cancer, she might overcome the traumatic events to which she was subject. Somehow telling one's story – making one's narrative public – not only becomes a path out of the experience (away from horror) but in placing it within the pool of cancer stories it no longer quite belongs to her, so that she might be 'allowed to forget' (1997: 242). And yet Stacey sets against this idea the equally tenable hypothesis that writing her book (which at one level *contains* and at another level *is* her story) might be a way of protecting herself against the impossibility of remembering; that, as far as she personally is concerned, her suffering cannot be 'for nothing'. It is notable that these conjectures (which Stacey does not resolve) appear both at the beginning and at the end of her book, separated by 200 or so pages of erudite analysis of cancer, its cultural meanings and representations. While she is wary of accepting any nostrums about the act of writing 'healing the wounds of life' (p. 23) she also says she feels safer with the text standing, as it were, between life and death. She fantasises that the text, in its relative permanence, might be an insurance against the return of cancer, or 'at least a textual trace of me will be left behind if I do end up dying of cancer' (1997: 24).

This raises at least two issues that are echoed in the work of other individuals writing about having cancer. The first concerns the work of *making art, or telling one's story*; the other concerns the relationship of the person to the work itself. For artists, the making of the work is itself seen as therapeutic, not in the sense of curing disease but in the sense of being engaged in life's rewards and tribulations. This was true for Jo Spence, who said, 'It is less about 'saving one's life' than about 'staying alive' (Spence 1995: 135). It also applied to Martha Hall, whose artist's books gave her a voice in the world and enabled her to make choices, which together she summed up as being 'about living' (Hall, 2003: 15); and for Elissa Aleshire who said of painting her self-portrait, 'the process healed me'.

The second issue concerns *the completed work as a product* of the author or artist, as summed up in the idea of leaving a trace behind you. This idea is mentioned by Arthur Frank, who in the Acknowledgements section of *The Wounded Storyteller*, speaks of his writing always being an attempt to 'leave behind traces of myself for my daughters' (1995: *xviii*). Martha Hall, too, saw her books as her legacy, as did Jo Spence her photographs. This implies more than particular works being identified with their authors: it raises the potential for stories or paintings to continue to do their work through their power to 're-enchant' the lives of other, suffering individuals. For example, the power of testimony to implicate others can be said to offer the capacity to heal

(Frank, 1995: 182). And yet it is all too tempting to hurry beyond the idea of the work as product, indeed as trace, to take up again questions about community and sharing. What books achieve in their material form is easily overlooked, which is less so for photographs and paintings. The linking of photography to death and mourning has often been commented upon (Barthes, 1982; Berger and Mohr, 1989; Harris, 2001), though less so the way that a person with serious illness might use photography or other artworks to figure ideas about their impending death (though see Creekmur, 1996). To paraphrase Benjamin, we might well ask about the work of illness in the age of mechanical reproduction, and will need to do so in the course of this chapter.

The question remains as to what it means to say that works of illness have the power to heal, and what remedy they might offer. What these authors and artists seem to be saying – based on their own experience – is that works enable one to live, even if not to survive. This is equally (perhaps especially) true when the person figures his or her whole way of living as style, in which case the work coalesces in the making and product together. This can be read in the account of her life and illness given by the political philosopher Gillian Rose – notably titled *Love's Work* – and in the story told by Anatole Broyard, who said that, 'only by insisting on your style can you keep from falling out of love with yourself as the illness attempts to diminish or disfigure you.' (1992: 25). What both of these authors offer in their texts are exemplars of their style, testimonies of their attitude to life, and affirmations of the erotic as a response to untimely death.

How might works of illness – as art – be any kind of remedy in the case of impending death? Schweizer (1997) makes a useful distinction between 'the remedy of art' and 'art as remedy' as labels for this kind of work. He draws upon different translations of Nietzsche's argument that 'As an aesthetic phenomenon, existence is still bearable for us, and art furnishes us with the eye and hand and above all the good conscience to be able to make such a phenomenon of ourselves' (Nietzsche, 2001: 104). By doing so, and by an analysis of Robert Lowell's poetry, Schweizer comes to the conclusion that art is not, nor can be a remedy any more than it can cure disease. What it has the potential to do is to console through providing a shape to suffering so that life might be lived in the best possible way; an ethical way, to use Frank's terminology. But that shape is still figurative, and the sense of cohesion that metaphors provide is in essence elusory. This is not to say that a sense of cohesion is unreal but that to take it prescriptively is to lose the tragedy at the core of the simile – art as remedy. Then one risks seeking in the work powers that presume a potential to heal, in whatever sense that word is to be taken.

The retention of a sense of tragedy – and facing up to this – will clearly depend upon the situation of the person at the time.

For those in remission, the recovery of the past might be a sort of narrative repair, though even in this case the idea that people are engaged only in putting right a disrupted biography seems too simple a description of their actions. In a reflection upon his seminal paper 'The genesis of chronic illness' Gareth Williams (2000) points out that his respondents (people with chronic rheumatoid arthritis) were not just asking the question 'why?' in relation to 'from what cause', but were also asking it in relation to the idea 'to what end or purpose?' The restoration of a sense of coherence came not only from piecing together possible causes of their illness, as in a repair of one's biography, but also in figuring a wider meaning that Williams refers to as the *telos* of the person's life. Where the illness is or has been more severe, and the future less certain, then the healing potential of narrative is more questionable. The suggestion that painting, making photographs and writing one's story can help is not to be denied. However, how these things help, what work is being done here, is less clear, not only in relation to the future but also to the past. The question of how – or whether – works of illness are redemptive demands some examination of what they do to the past and what role they serve in remembering and forgetting.

How Can You Redeem if You Cannot Represent?

It is useful to consider what happens when representation provides no remedy, or when its promise of redemption is already found wanting. There are two possibilities here; first, someone might feel that their suffering is beyond representation, or else they might have found that previous attempts to represent it have failed. In the first case failure is implied in the idea that it cannot be made public or communicated; in the second, that somehow the making of the work has not provided for the individual either the consolation or meaning that they thought it might have had. An example of the first case was given by the sociologist Barbara Rosenblum, who provided a rare discussion of this issue in a chapter titled 'I have begun the process of dying'. It is significant that she began her piece by stating the date on which she wrote, 'Today is the 7 January 1988. Two days ago, my doctor told me that I have between three and five months to live, maybe a little less' (1991: 239).

In fact, she was to die less than six weeks later. In that chapter Barbara Rosenblum, herself a writer about visual sociology, addressed an imaginary photographer who might want to document her experience of living with cancer in its terminal stage. She said that even with a detailed choice of pictures, and with accompanying interview, her subjectivity would be lost in the transformation of her words into text. She went on to consider whether having a tape-recording of her voice, something that captured its rhythms and cadences, might help. She said that, after a lifetime of writing, ' … only now do I understand anything at all about how the human voice makes sound and speaks. Words-as-text without the sound of my voice are now, for me, dead language.' (1991: 242)

And while the sound of her voice would help express her subjectivity it would not capture the oscillation of her emotional life that, she said, does not easily yield to expression. To agree to such an interview would be limited because:

> The camera, by its very nature, demands exposure, that I open to it. Subjectivity, by its nature, demands that I shut everything and everyone out, so I can hear myself. I find myself placed squarely in a contradiction between the objectifying nature of representation and the requirement of quiet and solitude in order successfully to stay alive to the subjectivity in myself.' (Rosenblum, 1991: 242-3).

This account, although not of suffering directly, is nevertheless about the conditions for its representation, and of the consequences of speaking or of not speaking about it. The reason for her not speaking and not being the subject of photography, she said, is the tendency to universalisation that would make her representative of the dying, a form of representation which relies on culturally common stereotypes. And the key absence in a photographic essay would be her own history, without which her words and her image would be prey to just those kinds of interpretations that Sontag (1978) was at pains to challenge in her analysis of metaphor and cancer. Lacking specificity but seeking universality an image can be reduced to a cultural cliché, becoming part of the spectacle that is comprised of the many and varied commodified images available in modern culture.

There are, therefore, two objections being made here, related to the two possibilities mentioned above. In the first case, there are the shortcomings of representation that would issue from the visual essay made by a third party, with all the dangers that attach to this kind of de-historicised rendition. There is no redemption here. In the second case, it is as if Rosenblum knew that such works might, if anything, upset the delicate balance of her day-to-day ways of coping. As a person knowledgeable about the research process, the need to preserve quiet and solitude was important to her as maintenance of a personal coherence threatened by an excess of interpretation that telling her story might necessitate. This is not a retreat from meaning but a movement away from explication, from articulating one's experience for others in ways that are amenable to record and analysis. What is being preserved here, I venture to suggest, is a subjectivity that is not easily talked about because it is fugitive. By fugitive I mean not only resistant to being denoted, but more positively, the retention of a way of being that is self-sustaining.

Rosenblum's presentation of this situation – of talk for the researcher – can be set against one that she does consider worth photographing, if it could be (or ever was) achieved. This is of her partner, Sandy (Sandra Butler), and herself in the night, singing together, or of Sandy reading to her from a book. In this case the world of silence is packed with meaning, even if seemingly beyond the analytic powers of the well-intentioned researcher. Whatever cannot be explained, still less shown directly, might nevertheless be alluded to elsewhere, in this relationship of people facing illness together. What Barbara Rosenblum offers in this possible photograph is a view of suffering understood by another – by her partner – so that the observer might 'see it' by virtue of it being addressed through the actions of this significant other. Indeed, in the account in her chapter, the description of this possible image is sufficient to convey something of this meaning to the reader. In effect, there is no account of suffering that does not contain some element of what Rosenblum has said she could not show, but to which she then alludes. The very silence that is held to be crucial in coping with the difficulties of serious illness is not over ridden when people speak of their illness. In contrast, it is somehow retained in the various stories that they tell, either to fellow sufferers or to researchers who ask about their experience.

However, we know that Barbara Rosenblum did speak of her illness to friends, through her letters, some of which were published after her death. In one of these letters, written eight months before she died, she says:

> I am committed to sharing this process with you, to make it more intelligible, more clear, and more real…To lessen my feelings of isolation. To connect with friends. To tell the truth, no matter how painful that truth may be. (in Butler and Rosenblum, 1994: 125).

Does this excerpt suggest that the issue of silence is merely a matter of keeping quiet about one's illness to strangers or researchers? In one sense, yes, because there are things that Barbara Rosenblum tries and wants to tell to friends that she does not wish to share with strangers. However, it is more than this because she implies that there are things that cannot be communicated even if, she says, the researcher could photograph her 'swollen stomach, bursting with its enlarged liver and liquids that are dammed up and not flowing properly' (1991: 242). These are the kinds of details – 'the painful truths' – that are shared with friends in her letters to them. One must suppose then, that specifying these details alone is insufficient for communicating her subjectivity, and that something else in the way she voices her illness to her friends makes for this important difference.

Not all painful truths can be told. Even for artists who have made work relating to being diagnosed with cancer, there appears to be limits to what they are either able or willing to tell. Eight years after her first treatment for breast cancer Jo Spence was diagnosed with leukaemia. This presented her with a new and apparently unresolvable dilemma:

> How do you make leukaemia visible? Well, how do you? It's an impossibility. It's what I went through before – a crisis of representation. I actually haven't got much to say at the moment. I'm dealing with an illness that is almost impossible to represent. I have not the faintest idea how to represent leukaemia except for how I feel about it. (Spence 1995: 215).

In spite of this difficulty, Jo Spence was involved in making representations of her illness experience ('The Final Project') while also collaborating with Terry Dennett on 'The Crisis Project: Scenes of the Crime'. In this series she and Dennett juxtaposed (amongst other works) photographs from her cancer project with those he had taken in London of places like disused doctor's surgeries. This work generalised her illness in a new way, but one consistent with her earlier attempts to produce a critical interruption to everyday representations of health care delivery in the UK. As she said of this series of photographs at the time, 'Not only does it celebrate, but it also mourns, accuses and attempts to heal'. (1995: 219). It is noteworthy that the ideas of mourning and healing are introduced explicitly here, which draw attention away from the other important feature relating to accusation. The accusatory aspect of this work is what it shares with activist art, showing how Spence continued to use naturalistic pictures as a way of making 'a historical deposit that can be discursively manipulated and re-animated' (Roberts, 1998: 213). However, the idea of 'mourning for what is lost' suggests a different view of the past in these pictures, inevitably coloured by what was happening to her own history as she came near to the end of her life. This raises an important distinction that we will need to pursue in a moment, concerning different ways of representing the past, particularly as the site of trauma in illness and also the field of redemptive art, if and where this is possible.

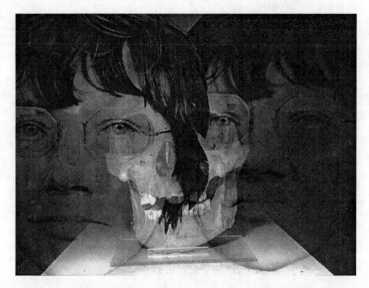

Figure 8. *Jo Spence "Looking Death in the Eye", The Final Project, 1991,*
Courtesy Terry Dennett, The Jo Spence Memorial Archive, London.

'The Final Project' series was never completed. It did, however, produce
several re-workings of older material and new photographs that made use of
various props relating to mortality. Spence believed that props were necessary
because bodily changes, the result of cancer, made it physically and
aesthetically difficult for her to use herself as a model as she did when making
the 'Picture of Health' photographs some years earlier. Nevertheless, she
retained the use of interruption as a device for making political statements
about her subject matter. One of the images shown here juxtaposes the
unexpected in order to make points about confronting death. Figure 8 is a
composite of Spence's face and a skull ('Looking death in the eye'). In an
accompanying series of photographs (titled 'Decay') Spence expressed an
acceptance of the inevitability of her death by depicting her face and body as
made of natural materials (e.g. leaves, rocks) that were in the process of
decomposition or disintegration. (See Fig 9). These latter pictures, though
derived from phototheatre, suggest that Spence was rehearsing not the past,
but the future; her own demise. And unlike her earlier photographs that had
challenged the situation of women with breast cancer and their treatment,
these pictures have an acceptance, a coming-to-terms that departs from
sublimity towards an older aesthetic. If there is a silence here it is one that

attains a positivity in its evocation of the long silence of death, not the pain of suffering that cannot adequately be spoken about. The question raised is how these pictures differ from her earlier ones, and whether they bear differently upon the wider question of whether and how works of illness might be redemptive.

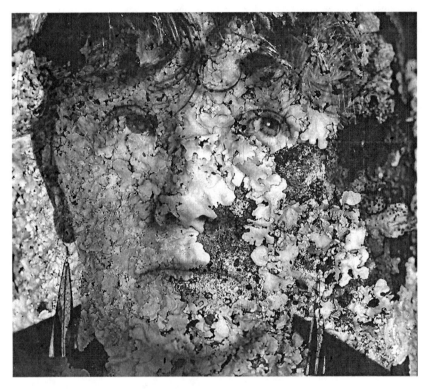

Figure 9. *Jo Spence "Decaying Face", The Final Project, 1991,*
Courtesy Terry Dennett, The Jo Spence Memorial Archive, London.

Compared to Jo Spence, Martha Hall was faced by a rather different dilemma. This related to the anxieties surrounding her treatment and prognosis of breast cancer, though she too realised that her illness was terminal. In spite of that, (maybe, by virtue of it) she continued to produce artist's books until the end of her life. The image shown here (see Fig. 10) is one of these, a book titled *Jane, with Wings* (January 2001), a square multilayered folding structure, 6 ½" x 6 ½" x 1 ¼", of hand-made paper that incorporates hair, thread, and linen. The book's spare text is printed using an Inkjet printer. To read this book is, perhaps above all, to learn to handle it. Its outer covering is a box covered with textured and hand-printed paper. A black polished stone functions as a handle or 'knob' for lifting the red cover of the black box. The book is a series of nested pages, all with origami-like folding, some made of card, others made of tissue paper. The pages are dark red, black, or white. To read the words one has to handle the book very carefully, going deeper into the 'origami' folds so as not to tear the paper, unwrapping (not turning) the pages so as to read the words.

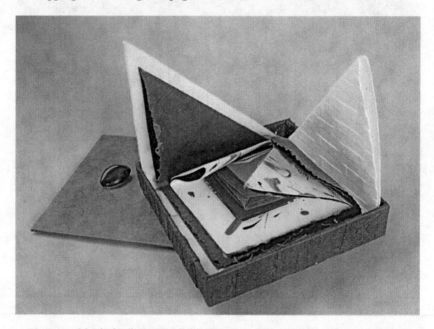

Figure 10*. Martha Hall, "Jane, with Wings", 2001, 6 ½ x 6 ½ x 1 ¼ inches, opens to 17 inches. Photograph by Dennis Griggs, Courtesy the George J. Mitchell Department of Special Collections & Archives, Bowdoin College Library, Brunswick, Maine.*

As with her other works, what is important is that the reader/viewer comes to *Jane, with Wings* in terms of its material form as well as in terms of the words written down. These tactile requirements are also signs relating the reader to the author, the healthy to the sick. For Hall speaks in her work not only to other women living with breast cancer but also to people free of disease. As she writes, 'People may not want to "touch" the topics I explore in my books; yet the books invite handling, touching, interaction.' (2003: 14). The lure of the work – which is its fascination – lies in its topic, its form, and its textures. The text of *Jane, with Wings* begins, 'There is pattern in the darkness – a crack in the middle, or on the edge'. In the subsequent pages she asks 'Do you see what you fear?' and further on, deeper into the folds, 'Close it away, the fear, close this page' then tells the reader 'You are not the one who is dying', an injunction that she does not need to see more, to know more, those things that Hall inevitably knows. The power of the book is in the physical unfolding, in the contiguous relation of revealed pages of text that speak of closing, hiding and ultimately of difference. Drawn into the centre of *Jane, with Wings* the reader is instructed that s/he is to close the book without knowing, without seeing.

Here is another example of silence, though this time the implication is that the artist 'could have said, might have shown', should she have wished. Like Rosenblum towards the end of her expected lifespan, Hall acknowledges a separation between the ill and the healthy. As with Spence's last works there is a sense of acceptance of fate, if not of melancholy. Or rather, Hall chooses to maintain at the core of her work a silence that she asks us to acknowledge; the impossibility of representation that means, ultimately, the impossibility of art being either remedy or redemption. This is not as it might first seem a counsel of despair. Rather, the message that enervates the piece is that Hall continues to make art in the face of tragedy, that she makes art in defiance of the inexorable moving forward of the calendar. In spite of this – or perhaps because of it – there is an important aspect here, to do with what is lost. This loss refers both to the past and to the future. Again like Rosenblum, Hall's later work continues to make public the experience of being a woman with breast cancer, but now does this by making a new turn, acknowledging the role of her art as self-sustaining. This sustenance is not remedial in a superficial sense, as we have seen; nor is it redemptive in the sense of rescuing the past. Instead, the message of the work lies in the refusal to seal up the wound, (her illness experience) which is not only a tear in her personal biography but threatens her separation from history. Problematising that separation would seem to be the final challenge for terminally ill artists and writers alike.

The Image and the Work

If works of illness can in any way be redemptive, then how is this possible? This is the question we need to ask, rather than one about whether any particular artist or individual felt their work to be so. Perhaps it was this latter question that Schweizer (1997) was asking, on the reasonable grounds that if art made under the shadow of illness might be redemptive, this should be detectable in its content. And yet, from what has already been established about the different aims and outcomes of art made in the cause of activism, or else in the course of witness, it is possible that works might be redemptive in more than one respect. For the purposes of this book, the question must be, under what conditions and in what way might works of illness save, make up for or fulfil pledges made? These three meanings of the word are worth repeating because they imply different ways of dealing with the exigencies of disease against the background of a given past and in the light of an uncertain future. This might be taken to imply that the past is that which is 'given', fixed, while the future is open and unknown. It might be said that for individuals with a terminal prognosis it is the future that appears increasingly certain – in its finitude – and the past a realm that has been made uncertain by the interruption of illness. That interruption – seen as a separation from history – presents the author/artist with the problem of rendering this in some way, either pictorially or in narrative, or both.

Whatever works of illness do in relation to the past they do not simply repair it. The use of the word 'simply' here implies that some kind of reconstruction might take place but it is not in essence a stitching back together of what has been disrupted by the onset of illness. The idea of the 'remission society' (Frank, 1991; 1995) is precisely that people are witness to their attempts to live the best life they can in the face of illness. This is because one of the tasks of witnessing is the obligation not to make forgetting a guiding principle. In contrast, the obligation upon the sick to get well involves at its centre this forgetting, this giving up of experiences that detract from the ongoingness of everyday life. To take an aesthetic attitude, to engage ascetically and imaginatively in order to depict and express the unrepresentable requires working with and from bodily feelings and memories, some of them traumatic. In short, it means working from images that make the past 'present in the present'. Jackie Stacey reported how 'an associative image, smell, sound or dream' (1998: 99) can evoke a sense of her embodied subjectivity that separates her from others and her previous sense of self (from her history), while Arthur Frank spoke of the 'tightening' in his body when certain words were spoken. That presence of a fragment of the past, or rather the willingness to give that image an aesthetic form is what makes works of illness relevant to questions of redemption.

The idea of images being 'worked from' in this way owes much to the writings of Walter Benjamin, who was 'ever prepared to place the image in the service of thought' (Abbas, 1989). Rather than using a visual metaphor of 'images as pictures', Benjamin emphasised the uncertainty and potential that lies in their having to reach out simultaneously to past and present. An image is not a visual or pictorial thing but 'that in which the has-been comes together in a flash with the Now to form a constellation' (Benjamin, cited in Weigel, 1996; 50). Nor, therefore, are images neutral devices, but are affect laden both in their power to repel and to attract, to provide the lure of fascination that is at the heart of works dealing with serious illness and impending death. Abbas (1989) emphasises Benjamin's conviction that images are potentially 'agents of historical understanding' in the way that they challenge our understanding of ourselves (our social selves). This is why Spence and Dennett deliberately made photographs that invite and interrupt the gaze of the viewer with the aim of provoking narrative to enable a re-working of breast cancer history. By challenging the viewer to give voice to the signified these art works create a temporal potential, concretising their moment of production into the image of history. About Spence's work it has been said:

> Recovering the past in the name of a non-emancipated present means recovering the past as part of a redemptive whole… [this] allows the marginal, remaindered and discreet to speak back from the past in all their significant insignificance, opening the past and *its* futures to the possible futures of the present. (Roberts, 1998: 33-34, emphasis in original).

If we refer this idea to a photograph such as '*I Framed my Breast for Posterity*' (see Figure 2) the idea of the 'possible futures of the present' is actualised not just by being 'talked out' but in being sustained within the tensions of the picture. To repeat a point made in another context, the aesthetic is not emptied by explanation, if only because it retains image-making potential. It is not just that images are historical but that, for Benjamin, history is imagistic: the past *and the future* are to be grasped through images. In their propensity to figure in this way images have a fabricating, potentially communicative and ultimately political role, especially at times of social change or personal crisis. From this perspective, they are no longer taken to give a full and unbiased representation of events (as with a realist treatment of memory) but rather re-present a displacement of experience (Abbas, 1989: 59).

How does this relate to works made by people who are seriously ill and perhaps near the end of their life? The modernist idea of the past is closely allied to the advent of scepticism and with that the notion of historical determinism. In his analysis of photographic practice John Berger (1991) has argued that the private photograph has the potential to recapture moments that are eroded in the relentless passage of historic time. Berger's argument is founded on the belief that to interrupt historical time is a revolutionary act, not least because it goes against the conflation of time and history that brooks no other sense of duration. These other senses are not limited to but contained in moments of reflection (Benjamin's *aura*), crisis, mourning and pleasure, to name but a few. These moments can provide, in their traces, the images that undo historical determinism, except that in a sceptical and commodified world these images are fugitive. This was because, as Berger says:

> Nevertheless a deep violence was done to subjective experience. And to argue that this is unimportant in comparison with the objective historical possibilities created is to miss the point, because, precisely, the modern anguished form of the distinction subjective/objective begins and develops with this violence.
>
> Today what surrounds the individual life can change more quickly than the brief sequences of that life itself. The timeless has been abolished, and history itself has become ephemerality. History no longer pays its respects to the dead: the dead are simply what it has passed through. (1991: 107).

For Berger, small acts of revolution are daily carried out by individuals everywhere who treasure photographs of loved ones, photographs with traces of meetings and partings that, in his words, 'look across history'. (This view of photography is somewhat different from Benjamin's in that it turns photography against the sceptical world that invented it – see Cavell, 1985). Berger's quote here is especially relevant to our discussion because it poses the issue of what it means to be torn from history by serious illness. On the one hand it means, where one's death is on the horizon, the threat of being disrespected, in the sense of 'being dead' even while one is 'becoming' so (Cassell, 1972). The fragmentation of one's biography is part of this, with all the concomitant traumas associated with disease and its treatment; associated with which there are images, bodily traces that at the time of crisis might be too painful to do other than live through. However, at a later, critical time, these might be made legible through, for example, the kinds of works we have been considering so far.

> "Anything about which one knows that one will soon not have it around becomes an image" (Benjamin). The image therefore, like some angel of interpretation with the traces of disappearance folded in its wings,

enables us to follow an experience which for various reasons cannot come to light. (Abbas, 1989: 54).

If one takes up this proposal, then for seriously ill people their whole life may become imagistic, and there is plenty of evidence that this can be so. Martha Hall's book *Jane, with Wings* is, in this sense, acting 'like some angel' in pointing to an experience that, in being made explicit in its silence, is demonstrably made present in its construction. Seen in this way, works of illness are revolutionary in their ability to show what we have lost, or might lose, even where they are not able to go further in saying how we might change things to alleviate distress. They are testimonies to a common human frailty and can be seen as a first step in sharing that experience with others.[5] In this way *Jane, with Wings* does not question history in the way that *Tattoo* does. In the latter book Martha Hall critically recalls her experience with 'a black man' to interrogate her social presumptions about black, tattooed men in the light of her exchange at the arts workshop. (However, we must remember that the books were made at different times; *Jane with Wings* was created in the shadow of Hall's illness being terminal.)

To take this point further, the photographs made by Jo Spence towards the end of her life, when she was dying from leukaemia, are different from those made when she underwent treatment for breast cancer. The redemptive potential of photographs like *Property of Jo Spence?* and *I Framed my Breast for Posterity* lies, as Roberts argues, in the reclaiming of the past in the name of a non-emancipated present. By comparison, the later pictures – particularly the Decay Series – are almost transcendent in their attempt to establish a view across history, but in a way that does not question it. These pictures are made through juxtaposition but with almost a positive aesthetic to them, so that they are tranquil, even beautiful. Not so much looked in the eye, death is surpassed but in a way that redeems not the past in the name of the present, but the past (Spence's past) in the name of the future. What is this past? At a personal level it is the idea of leaving a trace for one's friends and loved ones. It is also more than this in leaving a body of work – a legacy – that has its potential in the message that is passed on to others. Both Spence and Hall, for example, were explicit about their wish for their work to be their legacy, left for other women with cancer in particular.

We have here the beginnings of a differentiation of what might or might not be redeemed by works of illness. In terms of the recovery of the past, the

---

[5] Though see John Roberts's critique of Berger's views (Roberts, 1998, Chapter 7).

point has been made that, 'Memory implies a certain act of redemption. What is remembered has been saved from nothingness.' (Berger, 1991: 58). Stories and paintings, as well as photographs, can save 'from nothingness' the experiences that were borne by authors and artists in the times of their travails in the clinic and beyond. Facing and displacing horror is not merely a tactic in the making of a work, but at the very centre of conveying the idea of suffering and the way it has been borne. That is one kind of redemption, in which the past is *given its due*; testimony here redeems as a kind of pledge, a promise to be faithful to what occurred, to be constant to those who, unlike oneself, cannot (for whatever reason) tell the tale. As will be discussed in more detail below, there is also the redemption of the future in the present, in which what is saved (if that is the word) are virtual aspects of a life that will never be lived, that need to be imaginatively re-worked from their position in a historical imagination that had until then projected life along a linear track.

Images are not restricted to the past, but in the fragmentation of the present can arise with respect to possibilities previously unforeseen. In the light of his prognosis of terminal cancer Anatole Broyard wrote:

> As I look ahead, I feel like a man who has awakened from a long afternoon nap to find the evening stretched out before me. I'm reminded of D'Annuncio, The Italian poet, who said to a duchess he had just met at a party in Paris, "Come we will have a profound evening." Why not? I see the balance of my life – everything comes in images now – as a beautiful paisley shawl thrown over a grand piano. (1992: 7)

I cite this quotation more to illustrate that images are not restricted to the past, or do not only fuse the past with the present. This is, in any case, implied in the reading of Benjamin's writings about images as being revolutionary, with respect to change they might bring about in the future. However, works that aim at the redemption of the future (such as Spence's 'Decay' photographs) are not of this kind because they do not problematise illness in a political way; nor do they name loss or suffering, pointing to what they cannot change, expressing a melancholy that might be mistaken for resignation. In that, they are very different from the position that Broyard takes up in his attempt to live out the disruption to his history, outside as well as inside any representation he might make of it. Or to put it another way, he engages the images that arise as a result of his illness (he tells us) not just by writing about them but also by living them. He makes himself into an exemplar of the style that is expressed in his written account; it is an 'erotics of life' that steers his philosophy. He makes no attempt to redeem the past (for that is gone), or to redeem the future (for that might always be otherwise). Instead, it is the present that is gained or re-possessed by this style – life as lived is what is redeemed. Broyard expresses this thesis thus: ' I'm filled with desire – to live, to write to do everything. Desire itself is a kind of immortality' (1992: 4).

Compared to Broyard, Gillian Rose (who knew she would die of her cancer) offered a different philosophy – but a similar ethic – in her biography *Love's Work*. Specifically, about the act of writing she said, 'I must continue to write for the same reason I am always compelled to write, in sickness and in health: for otherwise I die deadly, but this way, by this work, I may die forward into the intensified agon of living.' (1995: 71).

Refusing the transcendental that blends the self and the future (in Spence's case the self and nature) Rose said of this approach:

> Existence is robbed of its weight, its gravity, when it is deprived of its agon. Instead of insinuating that illness may better prepare you for the earthly impossibilities, these enchiridons on Faith, Hope, and Love would condemn you to seek blissful, deathless, cosmic emptiness – the repose without the revel.
>
> I reach for my favourite whisky bottle and instruct my valetudinarian well-wishers to imbibe the shark's oil and Aloe Vera themselves. If I am to stay alive, I am bound to continue to get love wrong, all the time, but not to cease wooing, for that is my life affair, love's work. (1995: 98).

'Getting love wrong', but not to cease wooing, is not merely an affirmation of life but Rose's refusal to sublimate desire or to aestheticise herself. Rather would she make herself sublime, in being the performative focus of all that is unrepresentable about desire in suffering (Shaw, 2006).

In what sense can we think of living in this way as being sublime? (a topic to be taken up in more detail in the following chapter). Both Broyard and Rose reject the melancholia of loss associated with the disruption of 'life going on', with a biographical determinism whose repair means a return to the *status quo*. It is, in contrast, the catastrophe of 'things just going on' that Benjamin critiques, so that 'Redemption looks to the small fissures in the ongoing catastrophe' (Benjamin, cited in Abbas, 1989: 59). At first sight this appears contradictory to Lyotard's (1984) view of the sublime as arising from the horror of 'things going on' being brought to a stop. It would be reckless, if not insensitive, to say that this initial fear, especially in relation to serious and life-threatening illness, can be discounted. Rather, the act of redemption comes in the way that this fear is faced, in the response to the disruption to the 'ongoingness' of everyday life. To live for the present, therefore, is not to attempt a reconciliation of the past – one's former healthy life with life post-diagnosis. It is rather to say, 'This is life, and it is life as I live it here, now'. Just as the (postmodern) sublime spurns representations (and consolations) of an ethereal world, so too does it reject the 'healing' promised by the reconstruction of the past.

For Broyard and for Rose, what is redeemed in the indeterminacy of desire is a kind of self-possession, this 'dying forward' that in their life's work meant 'it is happening now'. In this they reject the melancholy that is normally associated with the Romantics, even though Broyard romanticises his illness in his account. In this they come close to Nietzsche's view that, 'If we convalescents still need art, it is another kind of art – a mocking, light, fleeting divinely untroubled, divinely artificial art that, like a bright flame, blazes into an unclouded sky!' (Nietzsche, 2001: 8). In his warning to stand above morality – but not just with the anxious stiffness of someone afraid of falling over – Neitzsche's example foreshadows a key moment in Broyard's attitude to serious illness. Some years beforehand, he had witnessed the decline and death of his father from cancer, an experience that he wrote about before he wrote about his own illness. Leaving the hospital after his father's death, he was watching a figure looking out from a hospital window when his feet slipped out from under him and he was about to fall, ' ... when without my willing it, my right foot shot backwards to brace me, and I poised there a second, one foot in front of the other, arms extended for balance like a tightrope walker, then I recovered myself. All at once I felt exhilarated. How alive I was, how quick ...' (Broyard, 1992: 127-128).

Beyond Redemption

It would seem that works of illness do not heal in the sense of cure, nor do they redeem in the sense of saving what has been lost. This is not to say that they do not have vital importance for their makers, for whom the need to write, the urge to paint or feeling compelled to make other kinds of work is life enhancing. They can serve as vehicles for coming to terms, for ways of re-entering the world of the healthy, as part of which there is the requirement that one be self-regarding. When Elissa Aleshire spoke of painting her self-portrait as 'a process that healed her', I take this to mean that what was healed was the existential wound that was opened by mastectomy and her experience of having breast cancer. This is self-possession regained in the act of making in the present. All of the individuals whose work has been shown or referred to so far have regarded the act of making as more than useful, indeed as necessary. Necessary, in the sense not only that it has served some wider purpose within the scheme of art, politics or literature, but also that the work *had* to be made – by them. There is, as we have seen, an allusion here to the idea of the requirement to witness what one has suffered, with the implication that something received – no matter how unwillingly – should be passed on. Whether this is 'for the good of others' (for those who will some day fall ill) or as a debt repaid to the past, including those who did not survive, is probably debatable case by case.

It is also certain that the skills that people already possessed when they fell ill provided the means of fabrication, and the professional worlds they still inhabit granted scope for dissemination. This is a hint of the more general need, shared with everybody, to continue one's work in order to get well again, or at least to live positively and usefully. However, this is not the same as the need to *figure* one's life in the shadow of serious illness, to render meaningful and to objectify the situation of those who suffer and face the prospect of an early death. What makes a work *of illness* 'stand up on its own' is not just that it has been made, which is a trace of an individual's survival; or even that it has been made well, an example of 'good art' or 'good scholarship'. Beyond the romance of tragedy and heroism and the scepticism of knowledge and modesty there is an acknowledgment of something that exceeds selves and social practice.

Seemingly, with this point, we are returned either to the unknown of mortality, or else to the vitality of life temporarily restored, each of these located in relation to melancholy or to the disruptive immediacy of the sublime. However, at the heart of works of illness that have exemplary form is more than the depiction of absence (or loss) and more than the communication of presence. It is that 'something' in the story we are hearing or in the picture we are viewing cannot be passed on (i.e. passed over). The message, then, is in the practice of telling and showing, not in the story content or what is or is not revealed on the canvas or the print. What can this possibly mean, and how might it be 'beyond redemption'?

No account or depiction deals with all of the experiences that the person has undergone. Any story of illness works to foster some forgetting as well as remembering. The idea that illness narratives 'tell all' is a fiction, albeit that they are often treated analytically as if they are complete accounts of what the author said, did and felt. What are glibly referred to as 'painful memories' can be thought of as images that still have the capacity to provoke a bodily tightening, that can invoke anxiety and fear. One of the tasks of narrative is to fabricate an account that involves not just the avoidance of certain memories, but the careful re-placing of images that help to anchor the account that is to be fostered. The use of 'critical images' as proposed by Benjamin would have precisely this function, so that their dialectical unfolding serves to narrate an experience that attains meaning at a political level, through a re-writing of history. This can happen at a critical time, which in this case means a time conducive to the image's re-appropriation. As well as this, the appearance of images relating to illness – that arise within suffering – occurs at times when the person might not be in a position to articulate them. And it is among these images that are to be found those that are painful and resistant to being remembered later on.

There is another, perhaps more important point that needs to be made in relation to images that are painful. Seen as traumatic, or resistant, they are viewed from the point of view of the narrator (in the present), for whom these are past. And yet for the person undergoing the experience at the time, which is passing into imagery, the hold of these images can be insistent to the point of making the sufferer mute. When Audre Lorde (1980: 22) spoke of the time of her illness, including 'a part of her flying like a big bird to the ceiling', she says that although she was in no state to decide, what she had to do was 'remember all the pieces'. As the writer of her story, she includes the idea of a time when the story could not be told; or rather she includes the idea of a position from which it could not be narrated. Put another way, Lorde is saying that her story was written by someone who had recovered from or survived illness; it was not written by someone who is suffering *now*. While this might seem an obvious comment to make it raises the question as to whether there are ever any 'illness narratives' as such; instead, there are stories or works by people who *have been* ill, or who *might become* ill in the future. Even in the case of stories written by ill people, works are always fabricated from a position that is aside from the images that comprise the experience of illness. To be otherwise would be to re-animate images of suffering, not transform them through the adoption of an ascetic distance.

Is this still to say little more than that illness narratives can only be written when people feel sufficiently distant from a painful experience? If so, this proposal fails to explain why people would ever write or paint their experiences at all; why not just let them fade away? The inadequacy of this proposal lies in the state of being compelled to tell one's story, or to make art in relation to one's experience. This urgency is, as we have seen, to do with the need to bear witness to what has been experienced, not only to speak about what one has seen or felt, but to speak as one who has seen and felt these things. In order to *speak as*, one has to *speak from* that position of pain and anxiety, which in the re-animation of images alone does not comprise a work at all, but rather the re-appearance in the person's body of past responses. This is not at all unusual but something we associate with talking about painful experiences or times of distress. These relocations both evoke and are enabled by sensuous images that concern perhaps a place and its descriptive features.

An analysis of a young woman telling about the time she was told of her mother's death describes how she switches from indirect speech (as narrator) to direct speech in quoting the people who said to her; 'Your mother died' (Young, 2000: 99). As recipient of this message she answers from the position of herself as a child, *'that's the thing that came into my head again'*, and *'I remember looking out and the tears being at the bottom of my eyes'*. As Young reports on the basis of the videotape of the interview, the woman at this point does indeed have tears in her eyes, and is effectively re-living the past not as narrator but from her position as a character in her life. The emotion of memory is made here 'not by making the past present to the narrator imaginatively, but by making the narrator present to the past corporeally' (Young, 2000: 102). It is for this reason – if for no other – that sufferers want to avoid re-tellings that not only 'bring back' the past, but make them, as narrators, *sensuously available to the past* in imagery.

This argument has been made in relation to 'slave narrative', using this as a model for other kinds of storytelling. Mitchell (1994) argues, on the basis of historic evidence, that slave narratives *per se* are impossible to write. These accounts are always written by ex-slaves, so that they are less about slavery than the movement from slavery to freedom. He compares them to accounts by survivors of events like the Holocaust, which involve the need not only to bear witness to the event but also to do this in ways that do not overwhelm the narrator. It is important, straight away, to draw a distinction between illness survivors and those people who survived the Holocaust. As already mentioned, the latter are removed in place and time, so that they are ex-inmates of camps in which they were held, whereas only some ill individuals can be regarded as part of the remission society. By comparison, Anatole Broyard and Martha Hall, for example, tell their stories from within an ongoing illness, and towards a certain (yet uncertain) future. And yet both of them, like other ill people, inhabit the world of the healthy and partake of it in order to make their works and to tell their story. What all of these individuals share is the potential for images to undo the narrative exercise so that, in the case of ill people, they are corporeally re-covered by their past. This can be provoked by the encouragement of imagery through description, often of detail. Citing Claude Lantzmann's film *Shoah*, Mitchell speaks of the voice-over dialogue that 'penetrates and probes like a surgeon searching out a hidden cancer'. This use of medical metaphor centres upon questions about the colour of the trucks in which people were transported to the camps:

"What color were the trucks?"

"What color? I don't remember! Perhaps green, I think. No. I can't say. I will tell you what happened, but don't ask me to go back in memory. I don't go back in memory. (Mitchell, 1994: 201).

Descriptions like these, often of visual detail, are imagistic in the sense that we have used the term, except that the painful images they provoke are not readily unfolded dialectically, are not transformed in the fabrication of a narrative or picture. They are the ones that people seek to forget because, as correlates of the corporeal responses they engender in the person, they not only stare back but are also re-animated in the process. It is this power of re-animation that is detected in visual details in pictures, so that objects stare back, and photographs come to haunt us. The implication here is that for ill people such images are traumatic, relating as they do to painful moments or those times when the whole order of their existence is put under threat. Works of illness, we might assume, bind these in the attempt to foster other images – not necessarily of recovery or health – but others that enable the experience of serious illness and its treatment to be told or shown in a composed yet truthful way.

However, to call these 'traumatic images' is still to discuss them from the position of the narrator who tells the story, here and now in the present. Once an image is made part of a story, or a story is built out from an image, or a semblance of that image is painted on a canvas, then it is made accessible either as object or position. Its power to make the person available to the past is diminished, if not entirely removed, although to speak from that position – to use direct speech as shown in the example of the young woman mentioned above – is always to risk that one is gripped by 'past' feelings, by the image itself.

This effect is amplified in the case of photographs that carry the trace of the event, which is not just the visual detail shown but also the evidence of it having happened. Consider the situation of being asked to look at photographs (taken by oneself) of the hospital ward in which one had spent time a month previously. Here a woman respondent gives her response to a picture of her hospital room (see Figure 11), showing the bed and associated medical technology:

Frustration. Frustration, particularly. And I'm feeling – I mean it's quite frightening – as well because of all the things that happened. When I first went into that room, I'd got pipes and tubes coming out of me all over the place. And so there were various restrictions – lack of food and where you can walk, and when you walk you drag all these things with you. And I just look at that now and I can remember every single pipe and tube. And the experience of having them taken out, something that quite (pause) ... well, it really hurt when they came out. (Radley and Taylor, 2003b)

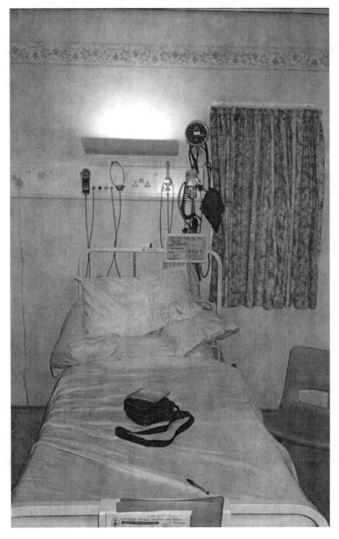

Figure 11. *Hospital bed, 2001. Copyright, Alan Radley.*

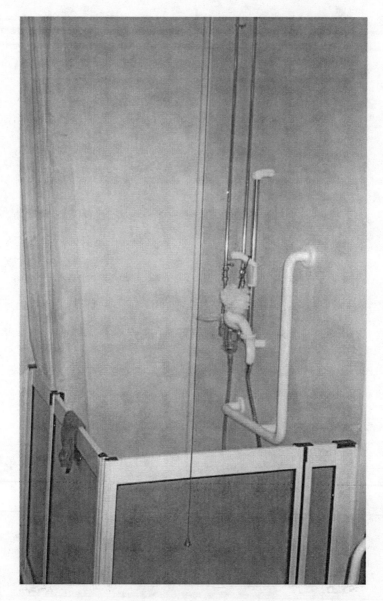

Figure 12. *Shower room, 2001. Copyright Alan Radley*

And in relation to a photograph of the shower room (see Figure 12):

> Again, the first thing that flashed into my mind is trying to shower in there. And trying to manoeuvre around all the pipes and the machines, the drip stand and things that I was carrying around. And the drainage bags. That's very vivid, just looking at that. I can just see myself trying to – and the very first time I actually showered there as well, because my husband was literally there having to hold things and help me wash my hair. (Radley and Taylor, 2003b)

Memories arising from the first, the bed area, were qualified with respect to her opening comment in the interview that she did not have a clear memory of the time at all. '*I think what stands out most tend to be the more – the impression of it all, really, the more negative memories, of being in there.*' This was said prior to the photographs being laid out, so that it can be taken to refer to what she understood as her spontaneous memories of the hospital stay. Viewing these photographs disrupts the separation of then and now, of the hospital and the home. Talking about them is both a commentary on what is there in front of her (what is shown now) and on what she recollects about them. The feelings she has about the pictures are felt there and then in the interview. (*And I'm feeling – I mean it's quite frightening – as well because of all the things that happened*). However, these emotions are made present through being related within accounts of what happened in the past (*When I first went into that room, I'd got pipes and tubes coming out of me all over the place. And I just look at that now and I can remember every single pipe and tube.*) Her reference to the act of looking at the photograph positions the feeling of fright as a 'now' reaction to what is portrayed. We do not take literally the idea that she can remember 'every single pipe and tube', but see this as a claim to the way in which looking at the pictures provides material to facilitate the justification of the overall feeling about the hospital experience. Speaking about the photographs involves not only talking about what they depict, but also making reference to how she is remembering. It is the 'effect' on her in the interview that justifies a photograph's relevance to the past. So she says that '*the first thing that flashed into my mind*' and '*that's very vivid, just looking at that. I can just see myself trying to...*'. These references to seeing oneself in that situation, as if the past were there in the present, are related to the strength of feeling that looking at the picture provokes. Note, however, that this is not simply a rhetorical device intended to persuade the interviewer of the relevance of the picture content. While it is certainly this too, in that she has been asked to justify her choice of photograph ('this is the most significant one because...'), the presence of the past in the interview is exemplified in her use of the present tense to talk about her reaction to what she is looking at.

The example of these photographs is useful in showing how, by 'drawing back' (the idea of the lure again), photographs make the present available to the past, so enabling the question:

> Suppose that the "other" spoke for herself, told her own story...? Suppose further that this "self" is a former self, not present to the speaker, but mediated and distanced by memory and autobiographical transformation? What would it mean for the *ekphrastic* object to speak of and for itself in a former time, from the standpoint of a present in which it is no longer an object, but has become a subject? (Mitchell, 1994: 184-5)

The "other" that would speak, in the context of illness, would be the ill person in the throes of suffering and treatment, of whom we get glimpses in accounts and pictures, in artist's books and in photographs. Rather than images of suffering being buried historical fragments, as Benjamin saw them, for ill people they agitate at the periphery of consciousness. For survivors of serious illness there are always reminders, like photographs or descriptions of horrific things that continue to haunt them. And it is this repeated attempt of the past – of a past 'ill self' – to draw the present (the person) in front of it that is at the heart of the need to transmute it through objectification. This 'ill self' is not a coherent subjectivity, (nor is it singular) but in its imagistic form has syncretic features that we associate with dreams or hallucination (Prosser, 2007).

The idea of images that agitate at the periphery, that can be provoked by talking about one's illness as well as by visiting certain places, talking with certain people, noting certain times and dates, demands, on a regular basis, not art work but repeated attention. Survivors of illness – perhaps like survivors of social terrors – are subject both to the torments of pain and the injunctions of witness that these images provoke. In that sense such images are fascinating, in their ability to draw and to repel. To be a survivor is not merely to be alive now, but to have passed through that experience then. And to have had that experience, or to apprehend it in others, is the *sine qua non* of witness and testimony. For Toni Morrison, other people's experience is an important element in writing her novels:

> Which is why the images that float around them – the remains, so to speak, at the archaeological site – surface first, and they surface so vividly and *so compellingly* that I acknowledge them as my route to a

reconstruction of a world, to an exploration of an interior life that was not written and to the revelation of a kind of truth. (Morrison, 1987: 115, emphasis added).

And she gives an example of 'tracking an image' by describing the act of writing what was then her forthcoming novel, *Beloved*:

I'm trying to write a particular kind of scene, and I see a corn on the cob. To "see" corn on the cob doesn't mean that it suddenly hovers; it only means that *it keeps coming back*. And in trying to figure out "What is all this corn doing?" I discover what it is doing. (1987: 117, emphasis added)

In these quotes Morrison emphasises that these source images 'compel', and that they 'keep coming back' so that the work of engaging them in a more satisfactory way requires an act of imagination, brought forth in the act of writing. The relevance of this example for illness experience is not just its illumination of aesthetic writing but also pinpointing the insistence of images in their way of addressing her. What compels and keeps coming back, she says, is not a symbol of corn as a separate object. Instead, it is her past,

And later on the summer we have an opportunity to eat corn, which is the one plant that I can distinguish from the others, and which is the harvest I like best; the others are the food that no child likes – the collards, the okra, the strong, violent vegetables that I would give a great deal for now. But I do like the corn because it's sweet, and because we all sit down to eat it, and it's finger food, and it's hot, and it's even good cold, and there are neighbours in, and there are uncles in, and it's easy, and it's nice. (Morrison, 1987: 118)

What Toni Morrison 'acknowledges as her route' to writing is her relationship to images like this, one that she allows to speak, as it were, from the past, and in which she rediscovers not 'herself' but a world of experience. It is that world that she renders in novel form. On this basis I suggest that individuals who have experienced serious illness need repeatedly to engage with these images, but in a more satisfactory way (to retain this working phraseology), and that this is at the centre of efforts to articulate what has been experienced. For some this need might be difficult to satisfy as they lack the skills, outlets and the opportunities to do this. For the people whose accounts and pictures I have discussed in this book, this 'more satisfactory way' is through writing, painting or photography – through *aesthetic work*. While remembering is at the centre of works of illness, they are not primarily an *aide memoir*, or route to the past. Like the illness narrative that is only a recounting, even a poem that 'seems like a snapshot' can result from a failure to realize the aim of making 'something imagined, not recalled' (Lowell, 1977). The work of 'making present' is more than a recounting of the past, is more than a remembering of something back there, at a distance. This point underlines the affirmation – made by all of the authors and artists under consideration here – they were, in a sense, *compelled* to write or to make art. This was not out of a need to neutralise the fascination of images: in contrast, they sought to preserve and enhance these in the course of making their works. This is because the key to showing what serious illness is about lies fundamentally in an aesthetic relationship, with all that this involves.

Drawn by Ghosts and Angels

In writing about their family and friends, Anatole Broyard, Jo Spence, Jackie Stacey and Gillian Rose look again at their past, searching for signs of weakness and strength in images made critical by the onset of cancer. Broyard had already written about his father's death from cancer; Spence had already been exploring her role as daughter in relation to her mother, trying on her dead mother's clothes to re-enact the past; Stacey explores a photograph of herself taken just before her diagnosis to see if the signs of cancer are there, the situation of the photograph made especially poignant by it being the end of a life where health, even when temporarily challenged, is basically assumed. And Rose explored, among other things, her life of love refracted through her love of life, prompted by the seriousness of her ovarian cancer. The images that compel are not strictly those concerning disease and its treatment, although these are likely to be central. Serious illness disrupts and fragments life, so that things or people believed to be quiescent – non-problematic – become issues. This includes aims not yet fulfilled, paths or pleasures not taken, obligations not satisfied. The disruption to the linearity of existence challenges not only the past, but also the future, the virtual lives that might have been led. And it disrupts the assumption that life is, in essence, a linear existence at any time.

In her autobiography, *Giving up the Ghost* (2004), the novelist Hilary Mantel describes her life around a long period of ill health extending from her student days until middle age. The condition that afflicted her for so long was endometriosis, exacerbated by the inability of doctors to diagnose it and to treat it effectively. The title of her book refers to Mantel's memories of people in her past, but also to people who are 'ghosts' because they are part of a life that, due to her illness, she never lived. What the title of the book also refers to is an act of acknowledgement; this is something achieved through writing the book and, the reader is told, through her moving house because the ghosts of her story are syncretically bound up with places and spaces, with ways of living.

Illness and its profound effects disrupted Mantel's life to the point where she says that the ghosts of the person she might have been – including mother to children never born - invaded the 'warp and weft' of her house. Mantel is explicit about the role of images in her work, and asserts the veracity of her memories due to 'their overwhelming sensory power'. She couples this with her principled belief in what it was like to be, for example, a young girl as compared to an adult, and the importance of writing the truth of that difference. In rejecting the (Benjamin's) notion of images of the past being somehow buried *back or over there*, she asserts their sensory nature to mean that they are more laid out *here*, alongside one another in an Augustinian 'spreading limitless room'. Therefore, while her story is a narrative, both outlining the course of events and reflecting upon them, it allows the images that come to her to animate her world, so that the sensory appellations are allowed space in her present surroundings. The spur to many of these images – or to them becoming critical and key to a re-appraisal of her life, is her illness and its effects. The realisation that she would never have children is the consequence of a total hysterectomy, in spite of which she describes in detail the domestic arrangements that resulted in her buying a house with seven bedrooms, two washing machines and two dishwashers. She asks the question, 'Who did she think was coming to stay?' unless it was the missing generation of her own daughter (she even gives her a name, 'Catriona'), bringing with her Mantel's 'green-eyed' grandchildren. Mantel concludes that the only thing to be done with 'the lost' is to 'write them into being' (2004:231).

What work is being done here, which is not about illness directly and yet all about the suffering that it goes on entailing? At one level we might consider it an integrative act of writing, in which Mantel's virtual life as a mother (including her unborn daughter) is woven into her past life to make a coherent story. As if that would be enough. For at another level this quotation reflects the imaginative work done to convey the semblances of possession that had been taken up by these virtual characters, that, by locating them in the present materiality of Mantel's house turns them into ghosts, into fellow dwellers alongside her. Animated in this way, staring back, they say to Mantel that she exists – ill and healthy – if not because of them, then *by virtue* of their existence. This does not mean that she writes them into being in order to be possessed by them, nor simply to dismiss them. Like Latour's (1998) angels in medieval religious paintings, Mantel's ghosts are misunderstood if they are interpreted either as objects or as hallucinations. They are key *mediators* of the work that is her story, a way of pointing away from either a copy-theory view of biographical events or a constructionist notion of invented selves, the social psychologism of today.

Just as we saw previously in relation to works of art in general, *Giving up the Ghost* has a message that it passes on, a message concerning how suffering is borne. But what does this work – this writing of one's life in the wake of illness – do for Mantel? Is it redemptive, and if so in what way? She speaks of writing – of her work – as an act of self re-possession that surpasses the specific locations that she might name, extending to the quality of the work itself. The aim is not a search for special sympathy, she says, because other people suffer worse without writing about their experiences. Instead, writing is a way of locating herself 'between the lines where the ghosts of meaning are', so that when she has set out enough words on the page she can feel she has 'a spine stiff enough to stand up in the wind' (2004: 223).

This phrase is reminiscent of Deleuze and Guattari's (1994) description of a work of art as something that can 'stand up by itself', so that one wonders whether Mantel is saying that art is no remedy, is insufficient a path to redemption. Reading her story further, one discovers that she gives up her ghosts by moving house, by literally dispossessing herself (and them) of the places where they abide. And yet the act of writing herself into being, that necessity, is beyond this. It is as if the work of writing, that must be done again and again, has meaning in its necessary repetition, in the fact that it is not redemptive nor perhaps ever could be.

How, though, to tie Hilary Mantel's experience of surgery for endometriosis with that of individuals diagnosed with life-threatening or fatal disease? While her illness was serious and devastating in its consequences, is it reasonable to say that she writes a story of survival? In an important sense this is the case, though among the survivors in the story are those aspects of Hilary Mantel that are maintained by the ghosts she describes, including her unborn children. What these ghosts put in question is what, of her, survives, and how has this come about? This would seem to be the puzzle that *Giving up the Ghost* seeks to convey. Rather than thinking of survival as a kind of partial or complete recovery from illness, or a tale of having cheated death, this view poses it as something else, putting it nearer to the idea of witness. Survival becomes a *con-dition* (not a pre-condition) of the need to re-examine how one arrived at this point, so that to be a survivor is to tell the tale, how best one can. This means that some patients say little, while others tell their stories and relatively few make art works.

To approach the reason why this is the case, we are led to the issue of trauma and memory. In an interesting take on this question, Caruth glosses Freud's writings by saying that trauma 'consists not only in having confronted death but in *having survived, precisely without knowing it*' (Caruth, 1996: 64, emphasis in the original). This 'not knowing' results in the need to repeat the trauma (to dream), and in an interpretation of such a dream, the words that awaken the dreamer – spoken by the other (or ghost) in the dream – are an instruction to the dreamer to survive by telling the story of the other's suffering. It is as if the images that speak – that compel in a sensory way – are an admonition to the person to witness a passage through suffering by repeating it. Not, it must be said, by *mere* repetition (as in a dream, or in thought), but in the act of taking it aside, by performing or saying it. And yet repetition is retained in this 'showing forth', in the fact that the images (the instances of suffering) must be given their due (they must be redeemed), by being given shape or voice, either directly in speech or else in tropes. At this apparently mundane level one can conjecture that Jo Spence 'saved her breast for posterity' every time she made a photograph of herself naked from the waist up. Just as Latour (1998) said of depictions of religious faith or love, works of illness are not exhausted in the showing or in the telling. There is no end to tales of witness because the work of survival is an aesthetic act whose re-showing, the making present again of witness, is the message that is being communicated.

Repetition is not about grasping that the person has almost died but, 'more fundamentally and enigmatically, the very attempt *to claim one's own survival*' (Caruth, 1996: 64, emphasis in the original). What this implies is that it is not mysterious death that is beyond representation here, but an awakening to life that such near death experiences provoke. Or more exactly, that some individuals awake not just from the trauma of serious illness but from *the sleep of good health*, that (as Hilary Mantel so aptly describes) can be peopled by ghosts. (To repeat, where ghosts are mediators, not spirits or things.) Such awakenings are not easily made the stuff of representation, in text or in paint or photography. When made the basis of works of illness their aim cannot only be to make life coherent, to repair or even to suggest the mysteries and muteness of suffering. As we saw earlier, such works of art – *works of illness* – bring the viewer/reader into presence, just as (but not 'just as') images bring the author/artist into the presence of the past. This special act of repetition, by which mediators are fabricated to allow others to trace back this passage from health to illness and (perhaps) back again, retains the need to return to and to leave these images.

To return to Toni Morrison's novel *Beloved*: Mitchell (1994: 203) has argued that the unspeakable events that occur in the novel require that it has at its centre a literal and physical ghost; this ghost must provide elaborate defences and mediations if these memories are to be passed on. In noting that the novel ends with the words, "It was not a story to pass on", Mitchell raises the question as to what these words mean. Is it a story that should not be shared or is it a story that one cannot "take a pass on"? The ambiguity about whether it is a story that should not be forgotten or not be remembered is something that can be ascribed to many works of illness, about which Jackie Stacey amongst others is very clear. In her various artist's books Martha Hall both shows and hides things by virtue of the folds and insertions that make up the pages and containers. As discussed already, in *Jane, with Wings* she makes a book that takes the reader on a journey that approaches its centre and then forbids looking, and returns the reader seemingly empty handed. There is no redemption here if we mean by this that the past (or the future) is somehow saved, or that a sense of self is rescued from a threat or horror that has been figured, if not named.

The message that is beyond redemption is perhaps just that: 'awake from the sleep of health'. This is consistent with Nietzsche's rejection of the search for truth as the guiding principle of art. He saw attempts to reconcile one's past or, worse still, the attempt to force the image of one's suffering on the world, as being examples of romantic pessimism. 'I am well aware', he said, 'of the advantages that my erratic health gives me over all burly minds' (Nietzsche, 2001: 6). Taking this view, to be beyond redemption is not a precipitation into nihilism but rather an affirmation of strength in the face of trial. It is only by virtue of an aesthetic response to tribulation that both existence and the world are rendered justifiable, a response that Nietzsche saw as compelling.

> Life – to us, that means constantly transforming all that we are into light and flame, and also all that wounds us; we simply *can do* no other. And as for illness: are we not almost tempted to ask whether we can do without it at all? (Nietzsche, 2001: 6, emphasis in original).

This does not mean that works that are conciliatory are not art, or that works that seek for unity and coherence are mere romanticism. What it does mean is that the search for an answer to the question of whether works of illness are redemptive requires a further question about when they can or should be.

To tackle this issue will take us back to where this book began, which is the context in which such works are displayed and debated.

Chapter 5

The Features of Horror

In her autobiography *Love's Work* Gillian Rose wrote about meeting, on a trip to New York, an elderly woman whom she came to call her 'Intelligent Angel'. At the time, Edna was a ninety-three year old woman who had contracted cancer of the face, as a result of which (or as a result of an earlier cancer, it is not clear) she wore a false nose. This nose was so lacking in its cosmetic function that Rose described it as something that 'could have come from a Christmas cracker'. What is interesting is that Rose tells of her reaction when Edna would call out to her to ask if she would mind if Edna 'were not to put on her nose'. 'By then, not only did I not notice the nose, but, if anything, I found the neat, oblong, black hole in her face even more appealing' (Rose, 1995: 4).

We might wonder at Rose's reaction to the sight of Edna's face without a nose, a sight that she says was 'even more appealing'. While many people today might not know of the stigma attaching to the loss of the nose, a symptom of syphilis, they would still be horrified at sitting down with someone without one. Gilman (1995) uses the novel *The Phantom of the Opera* to illustrate that the absence of the nose is horrific not only to others but also to Erik (the Phantom) himself, amplified through his love for a young woman, a love that is sullied by his ugliness. The dys-appearance of the nose in the context of the erotic makes for an especially unwelcome condition, one that threatens others willing to breach the boundaries between the sick and the healthy, the ugly and the beautiful.

Reading further on in Rose's book one realises that her encounter with Edna happened some years before her own diagnosis of ovarian cancer, from which she was to die. Writing the autobiography, in a condition of advanced disease, her earlier meeting with a woman she learns was diagnosed with cancer at the age of sixteen – and is still living at ninety-six – offers her food for thought. It is the consideration of Edna's way of life that leads Rose to call her an 'Intelligent Angel'. Could she have been alluding to the kind of mediating work that Edna did for her; not just an animated angel but a living one whose style of life, coupled with her longevity, pointed to a way of living successfully with disease? What Edna points to – and makes her gift to Rose – is the vision of possibly living for years alongside the presence of cancer.

And – we can wonder – how her impression of that absence of a nose might have changed in the light of her own illness. The nose of the woman whom Rose met is somehow unlikely to be the nose of the woman who has become a model for a way of living, a hope of how one might proceed under the shadow of serious illness.

I began this chapter with the story of the absent nose because it is an entry into the place of horror in serious illness. Horror is a word that refers both to a feeling and to its object, as in 'a horror'. It might be more accurate to say that horror is a reaction or response, so that the feelings associated with it depend upon the locus of what is dreaded and one's ability to move away from it. For example, in the case of people with cancer, the horror that might be felt is contingent upon one's diagnosis and what might or might not happen in the future. By comparison, the horror felt by someone seeing Edna without her nose, or seeing pictures of women with mastectomy scars, comes from the visible appearance of the marks of illness that is believed to lead to death. But as Gilman says, what also matters is the confluence of feelings of attraction and repulsion regarding what is desirable and what is not. To come face to face unexpectedly with 'the horrific' is to have one's 'readiness to encounter' (one's *extimations*) turned back quite involuntarily, and where these have symbolic meaning in terms of the marginalization of others, to then block these as a way of locating disease and ugliness 'out there'.

Because ill people are also part of the world of health – they partake of its culture – it is possible that their own feelings of horror are sensed through a screen that divides them from others. That screen, as described by Sontag (1978), is made of metaphor – metaphor that directs, blocks and diverts feeling in the course of making meaning. To find oneself on both sides of that screen at one time – say in the moment of being given a diagnosis – is critical in being formative of how people who are ill suffer the trauma of potentially fatal disease. Such critical moments might or might not be repeated, some might be avoidable and only some might involve the visible appearance of an object that could be called horrific. Unlike the idea of the nose that dys-appears, moments of horror for patients might not have a clear or tangible locus. We are tempted then to use terms like fear, anxiety and suffering in order to edge toward what is happening in these situations.

Why choose to discuss horror, or things associated with it, when much of illness is not normally thought of in this way? Or, when even serious illness is accepted as a mediated experience, discursively constructed? One reason is that, in relation to modern world, it is those diseases, in particular cancer, that remain unpredictable, their course uncertain except in the finality of death, their treatment invasive and sometimes painful, that are viewed as being symbolic of our mortality. In a different way AIDS/HIV is regarded as a disease of the modern world. The reason for discussing these diseases is that they are the ones about which individuals have written, as sufferers, as carers, or as medical practitioners (Cassell, 1991: Kleinman, 1988). They are the diseases that provoke fear today, that require making sense of, that remain challenges for medicine. However, it is not specific diseases that are at issue here, but the fact that serious disease, the uncertainty of its successful treatment and the ethics of living with illness provoke questions about how illness in general should be understood. And because modern medicine provides treatments that saves and extends life, so the journeys that people make as patients become the subject matter for others to heed, witness, or even enjoy.

Perhaps the most telling reason in this context is that suffering from a serious disease like cancer has been the background to many of the stories and artworks that are the subject of this book. One cannot discuss the 'aesthetics of illness' without attending to those aspects that are the subject of transformation. Taking up the topic of horror encourages an analysis that acknowledges that what is felt is tied up with what is shown, with what is seen; and that what is knowable about illness is subject to ways of showing that have a social form, that have a cultural history. In that respect modern images can be contrasted with the *ars moriendi* of the medieval world that instructed people in the 'art of dying' or with the images of martyrdom sanctioned by the church, in what Spivey (2001) has called 'horror by decree'. We should expect, in this historical movement from instruction to witnessing, a change in ways of depicting and ways of viewing, with different aims in mind and on canvas. However, we might also acknowledge the timeless human need to show suffering, and also to be sustained somehow by what we have seen.

The focus upon horror also brings centre stage aspects of illness that are arguably kept at the margins. This is not just because the healthy do not want to hear about them or to see them. Is also because those who have experienced the traumas of serious illness have needed to transmute them, have told them in ways that give them a form that makes them sensible, that achieves the necessary distance that makes these experiences things that can be shared. These matters are crucial to the making of aesthetic works relating to illness, whether these be stories or paintings. I want instead to explore how these things are made to matter (to matter differently), or else are removed from further scrutiny and neutralised in their effects.

Moments and Remnants

It is a feature of most accounts of serious or life-threatening illness that they begin at or near diagnosis. As a result, aspects of everyday life that went before this fateful moment are often only briefly described, so that they are effectively unavailable to the reader. The immediate mobilisation of medical treatment with its technical vocabulary and its promise of clinical intervention displaces the everyday world right from the beginning. For that reason, specific events are imbued with meaning deriving from the transmutation of the ordinary by the terrifying, often in the service of medical treatment. For example, Arthur Frank (1991) describes how, on returning to his hospital room during his treatment for cancer, he found a new sign below his name on his door that read 'lymphoma', a diagnosis of which he had not yet been told, and which proved to be wrong. Frank refers to this as 'colonization', the apogee of which was arguably the moment when, during chemotherapy, the nurse speaking to his wife referred to him as '*the seminoma in 53*', (his room number). What is terrifying here is not just the absence of care in the midst of technical assistance, but the opening of a door into a void of uncertainty.

In a similar vein, Jackie Stacey tells of the moment when, after surgery for the removal of an ovarian cyst, a doctor gave her the news that she would need further treatment in the form of chemotherapy:

> There is a moment or so's pause while the name of the treatment connects to the disease in my mind. A sudden shudder passes through my body as the realisation hits me.
> "Do you mean I have cancer?"
> "We're testing to see if the cyst was benign or malignant. I'm sorry . . . You may need three month's chemotherapy. The test results will be back in a couple of days."
> She leaves. I am left with the news. Alone, but surrounded by strangers. I don't think they planned it this way. I don't think they planned it at all. Perhaps that's the problem.
> But the nurses are furious. They had plans. They had plans to keep it quiet until more definite news came. They are agitated. This unexpected revelation by a doctor has thrown them off course; they are left to deal with the fall-out. They mutter to one another under their breath.
> I just make it down to the toilets, trailing the drip, hand on wound, surgical stockings on both legs. Away from those twenty or so strangers in front of whom I have just been given the worst news I could imagine. I look at myself in the mirror. 'Is this what a person with cancer looks like?' (1997: 105).

The void that opens up for Stacey is one she tries to fill – to give a 'face' to – by looking in the mirror. This void is presaged not by a realisation or by an image but by a bodily shudder (Latin, *horrere*). It is the moment in which the assumptions of time and space fall apart, a moment into which medicine steps immediately with its apparatuses and technologies. The hope of cure is premised upon the diagnosis of disease. But horror has entered *with* that moment, and its moment of entry is etched in the details of the circumstances in which it made its appearance. Arthur Frank says little about his feelings at the time of seeing the sign on his door saying 'Lymphoma', choosing instead to focus upon his relationships with medical staff. However, later on in his book he speaks of the memory of moments like this as being accompanied by a 'tightening of the body', the trace of a shudder; as I pointed out previously, this is a condition of being 'delivered to the past'. The action in these (and other) illness accounts continues in the plane of medicine, the discourse that from then on dominates the lives of those concerned. But at these moments something important has happened, something that is not eradicated by the progress of treatment or even, paradoxical as this might sound, by the deterioration of the person's condition. It is possible to come to terms with the prospect of death so that those moments of being given 'the worst news one could imagine' are drained of their violence. However, it is also not surprising to hear that this fear stays for a long time afterwards with many who are diagnosed and successfully treated for cancer. This is all the more reason to examine what it is that we mean by 'the horror' that makes its appearance at such times. For only by doing so can we examine its effects and its source as a root of works that are made to communicate illness experience, to 'problematise it as a work of freedom'. Implicit in this statement is the assumption that artworks and accounts of illness are grounded in this experience, though in what way and to what degree shapes the discussion to follow.

It is necessary here to give some thought to what is displaced in moments of crisis, not in the sense of matters having been lost (for then they are already transformed) but as powers that are now either out of reach, or which cannot be disposed of at will. This displacement involves not only disrupted work capacities and social contacts, which are the stuff of identity, but also the loss of aesthetic powers – the ability to contemplate beauty and to create space and time for 'frivolous' activity. This includes such things as the person's dreams, wishes and fancies. These are not 'mere fancies' but the taken-for-granted capacity to conjure the world as a fabulous, tragic or a poignant place. It is perhaps not surprising that this way of apprehending the world – essentially that of everyday aesthetics – is marginalised to the point of extinction just after hearing a diagnosis of serious disease. The sensed disintegration of life under these circumstances arises not so much from a splitting of plans and routines as from the altered significance of *everything* in one's world, where each fragment is drained of the totality of meaning that is the 'taken-for-grantedness' of everyday existence. It is in that sense that the idea of each object, person or event attains a separate weight of obligation as part of a past prior to diagnosis, deriving from its place in the order of things that led up to it, or its history. By 'obligation' I mean that even small things command attention; events in one's past that one has not thought about for many years return to show themselves, to insist on their continued relevance. In that sense, one of the losses sustained in serious illness comes from the double movement of the draining of meaning from 'things together' (one's life story) and their additive weight as objects that no longer have the assumptive frame that has, up to that point, connected them. When, at moments of crisis, people speak of their life 'passing before them like a film', it is not a coherent story that they watch, but the piling up of events of their past life all at once. The 'biographical disruption' that has been interpreted as occurring at these times (Bury, 1982) is not the cause but a feature of this condition, in which time and space – what matters, who matters, what plans to make or abandon – are in flux. Small things become remnants to which the symbolic world clings, like shreds of meaning. Life – if it is to be understood at these moments – is less a narrative than a palimpsest.

The two brief episodes quoted from the accounts of Arthur Frank and of Jackie Stacey suggest that these are moments of transition, in which horror inserts itself, or makes an appearance. This is not appearance in the sense of some object becoming visible, but an apprehension of awfulness, a feeling of dread that takes up the person concerned. At one level this is fear of disease, of what it might do to one's body, of the uncertainties of treatment and its effects, and ultimately of death itself. Susan Sontag wrote that, 'It is not suffering as such that is most deeply feared but suffering that degrades' (1991: 123). To understand this degradation of the person, one must see it not from the position of the healthy, but in terms of the incoherence that now forms its context. At these moments horror is not something that is referred to by a signifier but makes its appearance in and through objects and events. It inheres before it can be named, and does so across the boundary that separates the person from the world.

Two points can be brought together to throw light on horror and open up discussion of its role in the aesthetic realisation of illness experience. One concerns the idea of boundaries between the embodied self and the world; these are achieved and maintained through abjection – through our ability to separate and distance ourselves from our bodily excreta and from the body's decay. When this discriminatory power fails, or when we feel the shadow of its passing, the boundaries between self and decay (and death) are penetrated. It is at this moment that Kristeva has said that 'death infects life' (1982: 4) and the person becomes abject, suffering a condition that she describes as 'a terror that dissembles, a hatred that smiles' (1982: 11). What do we associate with the abject condition – that would throw us 'in a faint' into this terror? Not loss of health itself, but 'a wound with blood or pus, or the sickly, acrid smell of sweat, of decay' (1982: 3), things that do not *signify* or denote death (as would a flat ECG record) but 'as in true theatre...*show me* what I permanently thrust aside in order to live' (1982: 3, emphasis in original). Horror – in the form of the abject – is shown in things, which is another way of saying that it inheres, not in objects separate from us but across the boundaries of self and other. However, unlike an object, the abject is a condition, 'an imaginary uncanniness and real threat, [it] beckons to us and ends up engulfing us' (1982; 4).

The second point we need to marry with the first is the idea of separated objects that previously might have meant little but, in the face of serious disease and possible death, now become unavoidable. The significance of these objects derives not just from their symbolic meaning but also from their power to fix the person 'in their sight.' The idea of horror beckoning to us needs to be related back to the description of moments of crisis involving the return of small things to demand attention, the new significance of things that only hours before were the minutiae of life, or else formed part of the unquestioned progression of one's world. In the moment of its appearance for Arthur Frank the sign on his door that said 'lymphoma' stared at him ('commanded his attention'), just as when Jackie Stacey fled to the bathroom and looked in the mirror, what she saw was the face of a cancer patient reflected in a world that looked back at her. Such objects, to use Lacan's (1979) terminology, *gaze* at the person in a way that fragments the screen of symbolic structures. No longer does the person just observe the world, but, in a reverse movement, points (objects) in space gaze back at her or at him. This is a disturbance of space and time, a basic feature of the engulfment of the person in the abject state. While abjection associated with cancer has been described in terms of a disturbance of the relationship between body and self, bodies and others, and bodies and society (Waskul and van der Riet, 2002), the relationship of the person to his or her setting has been largely overlooked.

The passivity that patients feel at moments like these, reported in so many illness accounts, is only partially explained by the taking over of the person by medicine. It is not medical treatment alone that undermines aesthetic powers. Rather, medicine attaches its separate initiatives to the objectified concerns (about one's body, about life) that are symptomatic of loss of self and the alienation of the mundane. It is for this reason that existential concerns are inextricably linked to uncertainties within clinical and scientific practice (Adamson, 1997).

The power of the gaze that some objects acquire in the world of abjection (a totalising condition, not a property of things or selves) is amplified to the extent that these objects draw upon metaphorical associations with the disease in culture. Then metaphors of cancer or AIDS return to wound by connotation, grounded upon and referring back to the horror itself. For Emmanuel Dreuilhe, (1987) living with active AIDS, it was not the sight, through the endoscope, of the dark spots of Karposi's sarcoma on the mucosa of his bowel that frightened him. Instead, he said, what seized him with terror was a film showing cells magnified many times being 'invaded' and 'captured' by the HIV virus. At the time of writing he said that 'it haunts me still'.

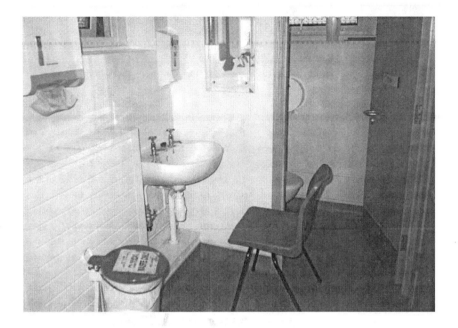

Figure 13. *Hospital bathroom. Copyright: Alan Radley, 2001*

Having made its intrusion, such terror leaves its trace even as the person works at re-joining, as far as is possible, the everyday world of the healthy. To illustrate this last point, consider a photograph (Figure 13) taken in hospital by a woman patient, some seven days after her abdominal surgery. She had been invited to take some pictures while recovering in hospital, and chose to photograph a bathroom on her ward. This is what she said about it:

> This one isn't a very nice picture for me. It has bad memories. I took this picture because I was in a bit of trouble one night – I think it was the second night after my operation. And (pause) I was struggling a little bit. Well, I wasn't too happy because I had already asked for assistance two or three times, and sort of been brushed aside, saying 'we'll come in a minute'. What it was, was that I was bleeding from one of my wounds, so to speak, and by the time they got round to seeing me I was in a bit of a state. In the end I tried to walk to the toilet myself – to the bathroom – and with all my pipes and my – what do you call it? – [*Interviewer*: drips] – drips, and of course I was trying to sort of change myself with all the pipes mixed up and I was getting into a bit of a state. So one of the

patients came in and saw me and said: 'Oh dear, you are in a bit of a state aren't you?' So she went to fetch one of the nurses and then she came to help me out. Now that was the really only bad feeling I had while I was in there, and I was really upset because I felt really alone then, you know, because there was nobody there to help me and a feeling of uselessness.

The photograph, chosen as most significant in depicting her stay in hospital, shows only objects and spaces that she experienced in the course of struggling with her leaking wound. We see no patients or nurses in the picture, no dressings or wounds, no drips or pipes. For us, as third parties, the image has a *forensic* quality to it, as if it pictured the scene of a crime (Benjamin, 1970). There are no horrors here for us. However, *for her*, this depiction was not neutral, because it had acquired its own gaze, so to speak. As a trace of the site of her misfortune, the photograph demanded she give shape to the suffering she underwent when frightened. The story she told on the basis of looking at this photograph served to hold that terror at bay, to distance it, to remember not 'the horror itself' but to make the story into a memory. One is reminded here of Janouch saying to Kafka: "The necessary condition for an image is sight", to which Kafka replied: "We photograph things in order to drive them out of our minds. My stories are a way of shutting my eyes". (quoted in Barthes 1982: 53).

I want to pick up on Kristeva's point that the abject is *shown*, not denoted, and to argue that its dissembling leaves traces that engage the aesthetic even as horrors make its deployment impossible. An aesthetics of illness – something eventually worked out – is premised upon the appearance of horror, is built upon the theatre of suffering that people with serious disease endure. Before exploring this further we need to turn over the concept of horror to place it in relation to the viewer as well as the sufferer, to examine the bodily spectacle as itself part of the gaze.

Staring Back and Looking Away

What those who have suffered bodily trauma often do not wish to show and what other people do not wish to see coalesce in the fact that many ill people live silently with the effects of serious disease. Before we can explore how portrayals of illness might break this silence, it is necessary to examine what it is that people are frightened of in depictions of the diseased or treated body. From what do we turn our eyes, from whom do we deny understanding beyond the pity that such pictures might evoke? It is imperative that we address this question because it strikes at the root of what portrayals of illness have to overcome. In order to examine this issue let us consider a specific image that is arguably difficult to look at.

There is a photograph of Dorothea Lynch (not reproduced here), taken by her partner, Eugene Richards, showing her lying in a hospital bed shortly after having undergone a mastectomy. This photograph is one of a number in a book chronicling her stay in hospital for treatment for breast cancer (Lynch and Richards, 1986). In the picture she is shown lying on her back, naked to the waist, a doctor holding up her bandaged left arm so that the sutured wound is open to view. There are bandages covering a drainage tube in her side. What do we see in this photograph? At once too much and too little. By too much I mean that we see, in a literal sense, the body uncovered and the body deformed – a bare breast and the gash where a breast once was. This is a difficult picture to look at, and one that probably many would be pleased to cover by the turn of the page. It is not horrific by some standards, and yet such images were forbidden to Lynch by the *American Cancer Society* when she contacted them following her diagnosis because 'books with pictures of cancer treatments aren't considered suitable for non-medical people'. (Lynch and Richards, 1986:16).

The 'unsuitability' of such pictures – the fact that they are restricted – also gives them a fascination, so that one looks to see, to see behind or to see more than one is normally able. Because of this, and because of Dorothea Lynch's partly clothed state and forced passivity, that looking soon feels intrusive and violent. It is a kind of looking without understanding that, in its frustration, draws the observer again and again to see what is not normally shown. However, the violence of the observer's gaze promotes (is repaid with) a power in the image so that it 'calls to' the eye, while at the same time returning its own gaze. In this it sets up a movement of attraction/repulsion where the person looks and looks away, seeing both 'too much' and 'too little'. As Elkins (1996) puts it, in these cases 'the object stares back', as all such photographs continue to do even after some time.

What happens when we turn away from an explicit depiction of this kind? In turning away the observer completes – in one particular way – the act of interpretation, inasmuch as it is developed at all. When we do this we remove the depiction from our view so that with its removal the 'difficulty' of its appearance is suppressed, if not entirely extinguished. In recognising this, we are also acknowledging that the pain and the imagination involved are our own, that we, as observers are caught up in the terrain that lies between the inexpressibility of pain and what is there pictured for us. The problem of the photograph of Dorothea Lynch – as with any photograph – is that we are used to reading these as if they were direct quotes from reality. Clearly, the photograph depicts Lynch's suffering and it would appear to be her pain that is at issue. And yet the form of this suffering is not simply given in the photograph, is not there to be read out from its patterning of light and shade. The apparently unmediated form of the photograph with its stark presentation of the mundane world depicts her pain at the site of the surgical cutting of her body. And yet the wound in itself is insufficient to explain the observer's reaction, because it signifies (by the presence of 'the healthy breast') the absence of the part of the body that was. It is the presentational form of the depiction that evokes the horror, not merely the revelation of what is removed or deformed. To react to a photograph 'with horror' is to respond not only to a visual image, but to register in that denial the other's suffering in one's bodily shudder. That shudder can be seen as the reciprocating aspect of the depiction – however unintended – that reveals the complicity of the observer in the situation of the sufferer. We do not turn from the depiction as such (there is no unmediated image), but from a depiction that exemplifies unbearable suffering. This points up a mode of representation that involves the 'setting forth' of the sufferer's situation. Such pictures do not 'refer away' to their significant object (pain) but are presentational in their standing as exemplars of this condition. These pictures are *with* the abject, so that we as observers become witness to the abjection of the other who is pictured.

From what has just been said, it is not the visual image that is unbearable, but the apprehension of suffering that is instantiated in the observer who lacks the imaginative framework within which this pain can be given form. The photographic depiction of suffering stands as an example of pain *silence*, in the sense that it is inarticulate without an imaginative framework to give it form. We might say, paradoxically, that such pictures evoke a silent scream in the observer, for whom this inarticulacy is made real. Unable to give form to the apprehension of suffering, the observer might have no recourse but to turn away. And this often works precisely because the depiction of a wound, unelaborated by accompanying narrative or other presentational format, is trapped by its inarticulateness into the moment of viewing. We look and are horrified; we turn away and the image and the feeling are gone. This does not mean that 'difficult' photographs are altogether forgettable. What is forgettable is a depiction that is presentationally inarticulate, or one that, through lack of narrative commentary, is condemned to being an instance, locked in time and space.

The reaction to the picturing of pain or to disfigurement associated with surgical treatment is therefore not comprehensible as a visual issue alone, for the simple reason that the powers of horror invoke the absent, the unseen.

What the observer turns away from is the depiction, (the *ab*-horrent) but does so in the cause of turning off the fears and anxiety that the image opens up. For if Kristeva is right that everyday sustenance of the self depends on abjection – on our abjecting that which is putrid, deathly – then these pictures threaten, even if only slightly, our powers of world-maintenance. It is not that difficult images lie outside of cultural schemes, and are incoherent, but that our social selves are premised upon the repression of desires and fears that enables us to assume the progression of the world, the narrativity of events. In this world images are made to serve the ends of cultural boundary marking, so that the beautiful and the ugly become markers for health and illness (Gilman, 1985). With that there emerges an aesthetic that rules in what kinds of pictures we should see and rules out those pictures that we should not.

Barthes refers to these cultural frameworks (which act as screens) as the *studium* of the picture, compared with the *punctum*, the term he used to designate the 'wound' or 'prick' that pierces the viewer. The *studium* is of the order of liking: 'what I can name cannot really prick me' (1982: 51). By comparison, the *punctum* shows 'no preference for morality and good taste' (1982: 43). Pictures of suffering are those where the presentation (in Barthes's terms, the *spectrum*) is dominated by the *punctum*, as in the wound left by Lynch's mastectomy. However, one must be careful not to conflate the idea of the *punctum* – inasmuch as this term is a useful one – with particular classes of objects, such as wounds, or genitalia. It is only in relation to the freedom to deploy cultural frameworks of looking that the idea of the *punctum* makes sense. For Barthes – who was concerned with what might be thought of as more ordinary photographs – the *punctum* is better thought of as an accident that pricks the viewer. In the case of difficult pictures the *spectrum* and the *punctum* are brought together in the wound. There is something literal about this display that 'gives it eyes' so that the gaze of the viewer is met, is lured, diverted. And for Barthes, the special quality of photographs is that they concern death; they are evidence of what was and what – with hindsight – adumbrates what will be. This gives photographs their fascination, no less the ones of Dorothea Lynch whom we learn would eventually die from her cancer.

'Difficult' images remain if they are deprived of frameworks that would enable the viewer to fashion a position in relation to them. This need not be a facile or comfortable position, but one that the artist/author might have fabricated for the viewer. In the case of Dorothea Lynch's treatment for breast cancer, her partner Eugene Richards (himself a professional photographer) presents this photo-essay in the context of Lynch's own diary.

This means that the photographs stand both as works in themselves and as illustrations of the text that refer to them. The narration around and with respect to the images releases each instance, each painful moment, from its time and space as it enables the viewer/reader to establish a position toward Lynch's illness experience. As we understand where, how and why things happened in her treatment – and in her actions – so the image of the mastectomy scar becomes bearable. That is, it becomes bearable for us insofar as we are able to comprehend how she bore it.

All this goes to show that picturing suffering is more than a matter of visual depiction, more than resemblance and revelation. What is at issue is the possibility of the observer sustaining a look, a look that is not overwhelmed by the stare of the object portrayed. This stare is the power of the image to overwhelm, to suffuse the observer with pity, horror or revulsion. Then, in moving away from them, these pictures can be designated 'abhorrent', and those who would look at or create them risk being called 'tasteless' or lacking in ethical direction. It is not the lack of health that is abhorrent, nor even the marks of disease in themselves, but the appearance of abjection, even in metonymic form, as wound, as death inducing, even perhaps as death defying.

Against this background we can begin to understand why speaking of aesthetics in the context of illness might seem (to some) both inappropriate and morally offensive. However, I want to argue that it is precisely this context that provides the necessary conditions for ill people to fashion accounts essential to the re-establishment of a sense of direction and coherence. Clearly, this means more than saying that people have to experience extremes of anxiety or suffering to write about it or to paint it. Instead, my claim is that it is in the chasm between the mundane and the terrifying that the 'horrors' of illness experience are forged. And it is the communication of these horrors, or rather the aesthetic form of this communication, that is essential to the symbolisation of the world of suffering that we term the 'illness account' or the 'work of illness'.

The Ordinariness of Horror

The idea of giving form to suffering suggests that, whenever this is achieved, then the situation of the observer can be alleviated. We can then look with understanding. However, a caveat is in order here. For this proposal is misleading to the extent that it suggests that formlessness is the only problem in the apprehension of horror. In fact, the presentation of the unwanted in the guise of the mundane (cloaked in ordinary objects) can actually heighten the sense of horror. The allusive portrayal of the unwanted and the unknown provides a form for their expression. In this situation, the conceptual or discursive form of a portrayal also provides its tangibility, its extensiveness out of the moment, so that (whether we wish it or no) the sense of that horror might be brought back to us at another time. It is in this way that both photographs and paintings have the power to shock (to make visible) and to narrate (to engage discursively through sign manipulation). As Sontag writes:

> Harrowing photographs do not inevitably lose their power to shock. But they are not much help if the task is to understand. Narratives can make us understand. Photographs do something else: they haunt us. (2003: 80).

However narrative – where it uses a descriptive mode – can also provide haunting passages. While horror might make itself known in the shudder of the ill person or even for an observer of the marks of disease, this response is communicable in the re-creation of the context in which it inheres. Abjection, the power of world-maintenance, can be taken aback by the re-surfacing of horror in those things that are quintessentially innocent, that are part of the assumptive world that we take for granted. Photographs, with their indexical quality, can provide what Barthes saw as the flatness of death, so that in response to someone who challenged him on this Barthes responds, 'As if the horror of Death were not precisely its platitude' (1982: 92). How can this be? An example might help to illustrate the point.

John Diamond wrote a regular column for *The Times* about living with cancer. He described how, prior to his operation for cancer of the tongue, the hospital dentist explained the use of a gel that he must rub on his gums once his salivary glands have been removed.

> 'With half my saliva gone that neutralising effect would be reduced and I'd need to rub the fluoride gel into my gums every night.
> "For how long?"
> "Oh, you know. For the rest of your life."' (1998: 84)

This brief excerpt is arresting because it indicates – without spelling out, without pointing – the way in which the treatment for disease would, unintentionally, further the penetration of illness into John Diamond's life. The *content* of the message is that this illness event will colour his whole future. The *form* of this exchange is such that the reader hears this as one who is momentarily delivered to John Diamond's past.

And how is achieved? The dentist's reply is almost off hand, so ordinary that it brings silently but unquestionably the presence of cancer before the reader. Not cancer as a disease, but cancer as a way of life, 'for the rest of your life'. The fact that it is conveyed by the use of reported speech is no accident; it pricks the reader rather like the *punctum* of a photograph.

At this point we are dealing with horrors communicated, not just with horrors suffered. The shudder – if there is one – is now with the viewer, the reader. How is this effect created in this instance? It is achieved by the appearance of the unthinkable in the guise of the innocuous – the reply made in the course of a dental examination. In this it shares something with the notice that simply informed (Arthur Frank), or the nurses who might have provided support (to Jackie Stacey). It is on the back of the ordinary – the mundane – that horror can make its presence known so subtly that the viewer or reader is taken by it before they can disown it. Pictures that show explicit suffering or violence are those from which the gaze may be averted almost immediately. They gaze back too openly to insinuate, too demandingly to be entertained. It is not our consideration they demand but our compliance, or submission. By comparison, horror makes its appearance more effectively in the context of the ordinary, and that this is not merely a matter of communication but also the way in which critical moments about illness are established for the persons concerned.

We need to explore this idea further to establish the point that the aesthetic is grounded in the sensuous. The aesthetic, in the form of accounts or paintings or photographs, is not the product of some ethereal sphere into which the author escapes from the pains of illness. It is instead a continuing encounter with the mundane, by which I mean a sphere of existence, not merely the effects of particular events.

The idea of horrors as being in part defined through their presentation in the context of the ordinary, or the unimpeachable, is not restricted to the sphere of illness. In her analysis of abjection, Kristeva asserts that horror can reach its apex when it interferes with what is life affirming:

> In the dark halls of the museum that is now what remains of Auschwitz, I see a heap of children's shoes, or something like that, something I have already seen elsewhere, under a Christmas tree, for instance, dolls I believe. (1982: 4)

It is significant that Kristeva says the shoes belonged to children, that they are heaped, almost formlessly ('something like that'), and that they resonate with an earlier *sighting* of 'dolls under a Christmas tree'. This is not a matter of connotation (not the *idea* of dolls in general), or of metaphor alone, but one of presentation. Horror makes its appearance here in its infection of space and in its disturbance of the moment, not in its inflection of words and concepts.

The appearance of horror is an aesthetic event, albeit a negative one. In its disturbance of the moment it puts before the person a sensuousness that invites or challenges that meaning be made, that explanations be given. But what explanation is there for horror? Does it need to be explained or merely (as if it were 'merely') conveyed, passed on? Such events are not only spontaneous ('they happen') but are also central to accounts in which terrible things (including experiences of illness and its treatment) occur. To convey them one needs to show them, and making the terrible appear in the guise of the innocuous is one way to achieve that effect.

A similar point was explored by Wittgenstein (1979) in his commentary on *The Golden Bough,* in which Frazer (1959) had given an account of a celebration made in parts of Scotland during the 17th century, the Beltane festival. After kindling a bonfire, around which the company danced and sang, a large cake was divided among those present. There was one particular piece which, whoever drew it, designated that person as the symbolic sacrificial victim. At this point the others caught hold of him and made a show of putting him into the fire, then laid him on the ground as if to quarter him, and, as long as the feast was still fresh in people's memory, spoke of him as if he were dead.

Wittgenstein argued that what is sinister about this account is not the history of it (i.e. that it truly represents something that once happened), nor that human suffering *per se* is implicated, but that,

> The fact that for the lots they use a cake has something especially terrible (almost like betrayal through a kiss) and that this does seem especially terrible to us is of central importance in our investigation of practices like these. (1979: 16e).

Questioning the experience of horror as a matter of interpretation, Wittgenstein alights precisely upon the idea that horror is significant through its mode of appearance, that it is *made more terrible by virtue of the way it is portrayed, not in the way that it is explained.* This is true of all such experiences, as Wittgenstein argued from a different perspective:

> I think one reason why the attempt to find an explanation is wrong is that we have only to put together in the right way what we *know*, without adding anything, and the satisfaction we are trying to get from the explanation comes of itself.

And here the explanation is not what satisfies us anyway. When Frazer begins by telling the story of the King of the Wood at Nemi, he does this in a tone which shows that something strange and terrible is happening here. And that is the answer to the question, "why is this happening?": Because it is terrible. In other words, what strikes us in the course of events as terrible, impressive, horrible, tragic etc, anything but trivial and insignificant, that is what gave birth to them. We can only *describe* and say that life is like that. (1979: 2e-3e, emphasis in original).

Using these ideas to underpin what I have already proposed, one can say that accounts of serious illness attain significance because they exemplify or portray a life (a 'world'), not because they explain the experience of treatment. The response that is evoked in the reader who comes to share in that world follows because, in Wittgenstein's words, '*we* impute it from an experience in ourselves' (1979: 16e, emphasis in the original). This is showing forth or 'seeing as', not just denoting what happened, when, where and in what order. Sociological analysis – whether of a modernist or post-modernist variety – certainly illuminates the development of the circumstances under which certain kinds of illness experience become possible, but its explanations cannot substitute (nor remove the need for) the portrayal of the suffering that it seeks to explain.

It is in the allusive portrayal of the unwanted and unknown that horror is to be grasped (e.g. in the presentation of extreme pain, ultimate despair, or death). Spelling it out (if one could) would belie the experience of horror as a 'terror that dissembles' (Kristeva, 1982). It fashions not just a meaning, but also a *world of being* into which the account (or the picture) admits us, as readers or viewers. That world is extensive across the sufferer's life, a totality that is at the centre of everything he or she does; (John Diamond says he wrote about his cancer because at the time he could think of nothing else). So, it is not the literal statement (or the denoted act) that he will have to rub gel into his gums for the rest of his life that is horrific. It is the apprehension of his experience of which this stands as but a sample, though a fragment that expresses the totality of his illness-world. Horrors are the stuff of elusive powers in human experience, made tangible in these accounts through the grasping of sensuous fragments that metaphorically express them.

To the extent that works of illness are designed to overcome – to work through – moments of terrors such as the ones described above, then they have as their 'material' the mundane in terms of which those feelings appeared. But we have seen that the presentational mode in which horror makes its appearance is also the establishment of an aesthetic, a sensuousness that may project the person into abjection. Whatever works of illness do – if they are designed to convey what it means to be abject – then they must convey this sense in a presentational mode, so that what made its appearance for the person concerned is also made to re-appear for us, as witnesses. Otherwise illness accounts that speak of abjection would not matter to the reader; they would be stories like any other, plots with beginnings and ends, heroes and villains. In his comment on Frazer's tale of the King of the Wood at Nemi, Wittgenstein makes the point that placing that account next to the phrase 'the majesty of death' shows that they are one. We might say, in similar terms, that the life of a person exemplified in their illness account or in their painting *is* what is meant by a phrase such as, 'rising in one's suffering' (Frank, 1998).

Of course, not all illness experience that involves unspoken terror results in a work of any kind, at least not one that is tangible, identifiable as a work of art. While accounts of illness written later on are able to give expressive form to inchoate experience, does this mean that the person is inevitably passive in the face of events and feelings when experiencing them? For example, patients undergoing treatment in hospital, involving complex and discomforting procedures and subject to all the uncertainties of outcome – what role do these things play in relation to the ordinary?

To illustrate this, consider another photograph taken by a woman who was in hospital for major abdominal surgery. When asked to picture her ward, she chose to photograph a notice board opposite her bed, on which the writing slanted downwards (see Figure 14).

She took the photograph she said, because it both made her smile and yet irritated her; in fact she said that 'it stared at me'. Two other patients made a similar comment about their chosen photographs – one a wall lamp ("a robot arm") and the other a floating balloon suspended from the end of a bed. While no horrors appeared to be associated with these items, they nevertheless came to signify a time of lying in bed unable to move, at the mercy of other sights and sounds associated with illness and suffering. The woman said that she tried not to look at other patients on the ward, to look away from things that reminded her of her situation. In that sense, the objects and spaces of the ward took on – or re-affirmed – their powers as part of the apparatus of medicine, which extends from the technologically advanced to the most mundane. Such objects are relatively easy to look away from, but they can also be looked at in a way that made the person's situation more bearable, and the use of photography helped in this regard (Radley and Taylor, 2003a). They can, in a sense, help the person to 'notice' what, in the words of Robert Lowell (1977) she 'cannot bear to look at.' How does someone in this situation notice rather than look at things? As well as looking away, there is a way of looking that already seems to draw upon the dissolution of boundaries associated with the abject state.

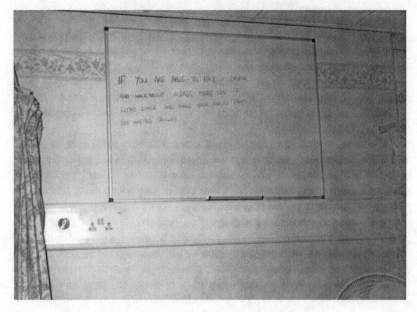

Figure 14. *Noticeboard. Copyright: Alan Radley, 2001*

In her commentary on Walter Benjamin's proposals about the mimetic capacity, Susan Buck-Morss (1992) argued that mimesis means more than 'becoming like' a feature of the world, be it person or thing, such as when a child becomes (in play) a windmill or a train. Such examples tend to suggest a conscious act, in which the subject re-makes the world through a kind of identification. Benjamin (1979) proposed the mimetic faculty to be much more extensive, primarily because it involves unconsciously determined similarities, constellations of resemblances that might or might not become figured in consciousness. This conception of mimesis has a modern variant in the work of Deleuze (1998), who speaks of the constellation of similarity as reaching a zone of proximity in which the 'I' can no longer distinguish itself from what it is becoming. To link this with the state of abjection is to see that the mimetic apprehension of horror is the condition for it later being transmuted, turned, named.

In a technological world mimesis is used to defend against the onslaught on the senses, to disempower the gaze, such as in the photographs of objects made by patients on the hospital ward. Technology as a tool extends human power, so that while it makes human beings more vulnerable (e.g. during surgery) so it 'produces a counter-need, to use technology as a protective shield against the cold order it creates' (Buck-Morss, 1992: 33). By mimetically becoming a patient upon whom such artefacts can work, the person dulls his or her senses against the stimuli of the medical setting and the interventions that it supports. The horrors of disease, the pains of treatment, the anguish of mortality are kept at bay by such an orientation. What we are dealing with then, in relation to the picturing of, say, a hospital ward and its contents is no less than a condition of *anaesthesia* that the mimetic capacity makes possible.

If this is true, then works of illness do not just figure suffering, give it meaning, but act so as to restore *the capacity to feel*. The aesthetic realised in works of illness is a sensuous act in the fullest meaning of the word.

Mimesis and Transmutation

It is because fear and horror are reported by people diagnosed with serious disease, as well as by those experiencing treatment in the context of uncertain outcome, that others understand what it means to be ill. By this I do not mean the 'fact' that horror is reported provides this possibility, but the recognition of its presence is the grounds for this understanding. Horror, as a reaction, often makes its appearance with practices that are exclusionary, so that a diagnosis or a labelling expels the person into a void of uncertainty, aloneness and ugliness – into an abject state. To communicate what it is like to be ill, it is necessary to describe for the healthy what it is like to be in this state, and to do this it is necessary to communicate horror. As already noted, horror is not a state that can be denoted, if only because it has the power of a gaze, that fascinates, draws and yet repels. The challenge set to those who make works of illness is to represent in a way that opposes the conservative aesthetics of health and beauty, for which sickness and ugliness go hand in hand. It is also to challenge those who see the duty of representation as being to police the boundaries of good taste. This challenge is not an idle one: it is necessary if serious illness is to be given a voice. It might seem strange to speak of illness as having a 'voice' when we are used to describing the ill in this way, where voice connotes actual speaking. But we are also concerned here with the communication of a state of being with which the ill person is identified, so that it is not some location at a distance that is being talked about, but a world that is being configured. This is not so far from the idea that the illness world is a life lived aesthetically: not the person's everyday life, but their life of illness, the fateful adventure that they did not seek but yet have to negotiate as best they can.

So, to speak of illness as being given a voice is to acknowledge that stories and pictures expressing it have, as an important quality, the power of fascination. As Adorno put it:

> Expression is the gaze of an art work. The language of expression is older than its significative counterpart; it is also unredeemed. It is as if art works were re-enacting the process through which the subject comes painfully into being. (1984: 165).

Aesthetically powerful works are texts or pictures that do more than command attention; they also, in this context, fashion a world of illness that has at its centre a transmutation of horror. A corollary of this is that there are narratives (and pictures) that have little or no aesthetic power, and this follows from their mode of representation. While this idea will be discussed more fully below, it is enough to say for the moment that such works are 'different from' rather than 'less than', and that this difference derives from the way that they denote their subject matter, rather than in the way that they evoke it.

The key to the issue of how individuals are able to represent their suffering lies in the fact that they are already possessed by it. Pain and suffering are conditions of incoherence and ultimately of abjection in which boundaries are not only dissolved within the self but between person and the world. Extreme pain and suffering involve an assimilation to space, the 'lure' of which involves a fundamental disturbance (Caillois, 1984). This is also mimesis, by which I do not mean a resemblance of this to that, as the term is used sometimes when speaking of picturing or copying the world. I want to emphasise a particular reading, which Ricoeur (1991) calls 'mimesis$_1$' to underline its condition of action and suffering as *already understood*.

Understood in this way, mimesis is not a cognitive operation of copying or deliberate position taking. Instead, it is a *semblance* such that subjects and ideas can be replaced or overlaid in a condition of 'standing for' each other. This means that where one aspect is sentient then it experiences a dissolving of its separateness into the other, the self into the dream, into the landscape. It is an experience of 'to become like', or 'to be as', as part of which the other aspect – the landscape for example – acquires powers (e.g. 'to see') in its turn. This double movement – that underlies the fall into incoherence during serious illness – is well expressed by Deleuze and Guattari as one in which, 'affects are precisely these nonhuman becomings of man, just as percepts are nonhuman landscapes of nature' (1994: 169). To illustrate this, Arthur Frank wrote that his cancer 'connected pain with night', qualifying this by saying that:

> I could write that at night in pain I came to know illness face to face. But this metaphor distorts the experience. However much I wanted to give illness a face – to give it any kind of coherence – it is not a presence. Giving illness a face, *a temptation enhanced by the dark*, only muddles things further. At night I faced only myself. (1991: 30, emphasis added).

Note the emphasised words by which Frank gives credence to the idea (proposed by Caillois) that, in these conditions of vulnerability, we are especially *tempted* by place, by the lure of the dark.

One condition for passing beyond abjection is to look *through* horror *with* the eyes of the landscape that mimesis makes possible. This is not to be confused with seeing the face of horror (as if this could be done). How is this special way of looking possible? In terms of works of illness we are talking about a fashioned landscape – one that is representational in being a screen that modulates and pacifies the horror of illness's gaze. But this is not available to people at diagnosis, or in the early stages of treatment, when the avoidance of horror – the clinging to the shreds of the mundane – is likely to be the primary goal. After surgery, for example, the mimetic mode offers the possibility of countering sensibility, of dulling the senses (Benjamin, 1970; Buck-Morss, 1992). As Audre Lorde said about the time just after her mastectomy:

> I was very anxious to go home. But I found also, and wouldn't admit at the time, that the very bland whiteness of the hospital which I railed against and hated so, was also a kind of protection, a welcome insulation within which I could continue to non-feel. It was an erotically blank environment within whose undifferentiated and undemanding and infantalizing walls I could continue to be emotionally vacant – psychic mush – without being required by myself or anyone to be anything else. (1980: 38).

Similarly, hospital patients speak of an irritated amusement brought about by the contemplation of objects that seem to 'stare at them' while they lie in their beds after surgery. (See notice board, Figure 14). These objects contrast with those that are cold and clinical, forbidding in their evocation of steel against the soft fragility of the ailing body. The mimetic stance offers a counter to feeling, a self-induced anaesthesia, and yet in the animation of things like the notice board it makes something else possible. This is the first inklings of feeling, of amusement and delight, as well as the first evidence of the power of mimesis to fashion contiguities with positive affect. What it shows is that the mimetic stance is active beyond horror, that whether or not positive affect is sought there is scope for reversals of incoherence in contiguous relationships where the landscape looks upon the person 'with affection'.

For Arthur Frank, in chronic pain due to a failure to diagnose cancer, this mimetic act occurred one night as he stood before a window in his home:

> Although I never discovered a formula for dealing with pain, I did manage to break through its incoherence one night before it abated. Making my way upstairs, I was stopped on the landing by the sight – the vision really – of a window. Outside the window I saw a tree, and the streetlight just beyond was casting the tree's reflection on the frosted glass. Here suddenly was beauty, found in the middle of a night that seemed to be only darkness and pain. Where we see the face of beauty, we are in our proper place, and all becomes coherent. (1991: 33)

Frank offers a small poem to this vision and then continues, 'I realized that if illness has a face, it could be the beauty of that light. But I did not see the face of illness in that window any more than I had seen it in the nightmares caused by the pain breaking through the sedative' (1991: 34). He explicitly denies that the view from the window was a (mere) metaphor, in that he says it was 'exactly what it was', a placing of an image in the place of a feeling. Not only does this image 'fail' to explain his pain, it 'fails' to reveal horror. However, we can take these supposed failures to be evidence of a new positivity, in which Frank finds himself again in the reflection of a gaze that emanates from outside. His description of this experience, given at a point later on in the book, supports this argument:

> In that frosted window I saw myself. Not the self I see in a mirror, but a world I am so completely a part of that it too is myself. The sight allowed me to exist outside my body's pain and at the same time to see why that pain was part of the same world as the window, as necessary to that world as the window's beauty was. (1991: 141).

What this excerpt suggests is that this vision made possible a transmutation of suffering, so that Frank's pain was given what one might call 'another shape', one that he could re-appropriate later and work on. It is the *features of horror*, rather than its face, which are given in presentations like these. It might be said that, rather than looking through the eyes of pain, Frank looked *with* the eyes of beauty, as if to counter horror. And yet this image is, by his admission, soaked in pain, so that suffering re-appears in a different guise, not cleansed but somehow transformed. What then continues to appear to others as 'horrific' (the prospect of cancer, its treatment, the uncertainty of recovery) became for Frank a portal swung back to allow entry into a different view of himself in the world. In terms too simple, yet I think appropriate, the image on the staircase for which suffering is a necessary precondition became for Frank a primitive screen to deflect the gaze of horror. And in becoming this, what for the healthy appears as the ugliness of illness contained for Frank the possibility of a sort of redemption.

Of course, the excerpts cited from Frank's writing are taken from an essay that is, by my terms, a work of illness in itself. In his essay he not only describes what befell him during his two illnesses – especially his misdiagnosed testicular cancer – but he also attempts to give expression to the feelings and circumstances in which he moved from being in the grip of pain (and suffering) to one where he could bear witness to what had happened to him. It is necessary to distinguish the different possible readings that we can take from his work. One concerns the essay as a story, one that can be discussed in terms of narrative forms and the dialogic context – this is Frank's own developed position (Frank, 1995; 2004). The other – which I am entertaining here – regards such work as a repository of images, or features. These images can be dug out from the seams of narrative and examined for their historical function, as clues to the way that the story came about. I use the words 'historical function' in order to indicate that such images 'worked' for Frank *before* he wrote his essay, before he worked them into a story making a narrative screen through which his cancer is made to appear for us, the readers. As the excerpts indicate, it is the affective harmony of his vision on the staircase landing that show the function of these images to be aesthetic, through which is created an erotics of place.

Giving Shape to Illness

The idea of 'needing to look death in the face', yet not to embrace it too easily is a task for recovery, one that Audre Lorde said was constantly being sidelined by the practical demands of 'hurting too much'. She asked, in relation to this, 'What posture do I take, literally, with my physical self?' (Lorde, 1980: 39).

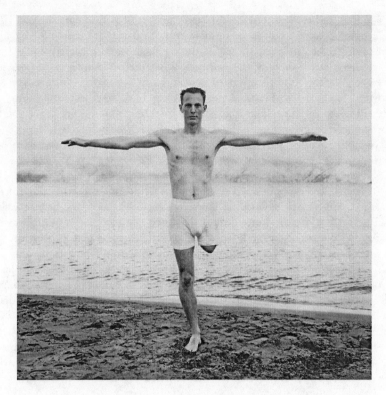

Figure 15. *Ian Robertson, "Stefan Wahrlich", 1998.*
Courtesy R. and J. Watson Trust and the Cancer Society of New Zealand.

To help address this issue of posture and pain, examine the photograph for
an exhibition of words and pictures entitled 'I Feel Lucky' (Ogonowska-
Coates and Robertson, 1998). (See Figure 15). This exhibition consisted of
interviews and portraits of cancer survivors and included this image of a
young man – Stefan Wahrlich – standing on a beach with a backdrop of sea
and distant hills. He faces directly to camera, wearing only a pair of shorts,
arms outstretched and standing on one leg. The other leg is visible only as a
stump below his shorts, where it was removed as treatment for cancer of the
bone. In the exhibition this image was displayed above a brief commentary
explaining the background to his illness and his reactions to it.

At one level, the photographic form of this image is a record, an instance.
And yet the pose is counterfactual by virtue of it both revealing the absent leg
and defying that absence. This is a pose that is more than an alignment with

what Goffman (1976) called 'schedules' for being pictured in particular situations. However, photo-schedules for cancer patients (especially with one leg amputated) do not exist, so that the portrayal in this image must make use of, in order to transcend, some of the conventions by which individuals might be pictured standing on a beach. In Stefan Wahrlich's case, the image conveys meaning through this transcendence, wherein the achievement of balance, of the symmetry of his arms, overcomes the literal instability that must follow from his having had a leg amputated. In this picture he does not just pose for the camera, but asserts his position *vis-à-vis the world* and the camera/observer. This image is coherent and expressive, in that it exemplifies a world of 'suffering-as-borne'. It also achieves meaning through figurative portrayal, which is the condition for any work to be deemed 'artistic'.

As viewers, we might compare it with the unity shown in Leonardo's figure of a man inscribed within a circle, a pose that Stefan Wahrlich's portrait suggests. Certainly cultural forms guide the making and the reading of images; the history of art shows that there were conventions in Renaissance painting and sculpture about picturing the body in terms of the disposition of the limbs. These concerned the way that the pose of the body was portrayed ('contrapposto') so as to indicate feeling, where twisting of the figure expressed suffering, as in the figure of Christ on the cross (Elkins, 1999).

In order to try to analyse this photograph further, we need to see such work as involving both artist and model, for it is in the form of the pose captured by the camera that Stefan Wahrlich's world is to be apprehended. Instead of seeing it as a 'mere pose', we should recognise its mimetic power as a kind of static dance, in that the various countervailing tensions are held in a dynamic equilibrium in his balancing posture. Considered as a (static) dance what was originally an inchoate response to disease and its treatment is made visible; considered as the capturing of that dance, the photograph becomes the artefactual structure of this communicable act. We can understand Stefan Wahrlich's 'dance' as one that *gives shape* to his world of 'suffering-as-borne', that says 'this, *precisely, this,* is how it is'. In that sense it is his answer to Lorde's question, 'what posture should I take?' though not just considered literally. Where Lorde was concerned with the mundane aftermath of surgery, Stefan Warlich's image is similar to Frank's vision in its power to imagine pain.

In the case of this picture the mimetic stance is actually sidelined for us – the viewers – by a framing that privileges our point of view. A different version of events is provided by entertaining the idea that Stefan Wahrlich makes himself an object of vision within the landscape, configured by his posture *vis-a-vis* the landscape. Otherwise – holding merely to the idea that he is a pictured subject – we render him the object of scrutiny, when in truth he chose this pose, made the camera witness to the look he directs at the lens.

Feature-placing and Fortuitous Fragments

At this point I am making my argument beneath or before representation, if that is possible. What I mean here is that I am having to speak of a place which is given to us in clues by writers such as Arthur Frank but found already in our own experience, without which it could not be known. In consequence, we grasp it rather than deduce it from what is given, and cannot adequately justify it through explanation. Works (stories, pictures) transform these images and feelings so as to present them together, if not always coherently, and provide that narrative basis for the modulated contemplation of what serious illness involves. And in the end, whatever the experience, it can only be shared through some kind of representation. But of what kind? And at what level?

Unlike narratives, poems and paintings remain closer to the made up stage. Quite literally, it is possible to sketch the moment, to try to capture in a few lines the feeling of a fragment of time. Consider Figure 16, titled *Steeple,* a drawing by Robert Pope made with charcoal on paper. This shows a woman patient sitting on her hospital bed staring out of the window. Beyond is a view of a church steeple. In the foreground is an IV line and bag, to which the woman is attached. Like many of Pope's drawings this one evokes a sense of waiting, of the person being suspended between illness and health in the uncertainty of outcome.

Looking at this picture I am filled with a sense of depression, the heavy feeling of dread that comes of deep uncertainty and forced passivity. It is not the content alone that carries expressive meaning in this drawing but the way that the charcoal medium deploys light and shade to create a sense of inactivity. This, the inactivity of illness, is almost a palpable presence here, and realised in the light/shading that blurs the edges between the people and the hospital surroundings. Just as the patient must occupy the room – attached to the line – so the room with its medical technology will occupy the patient. Her stare fills – if it can – a space and time that extends onwards for who knows how long, and with what end? There is sadness here and isolation. And this is horrible.

One is reminded of the charcoal drawings of the German artist Kathe Kollwitz, who often drew poor and ailing people (especially women) in the context of deprived surroundings, so that the darkness of the setting permeated the figures, setting a mood of despair. The sense of space/time in Pope's drawings also evokes the menacing piazzas in the paintings of de Cirico, of late afternoon light slanting into a room, the hopes of the day gradually being eroded by the advancing dusk. For anyone who has been in hospital with serious disease, these pictures are able to bring back that sense of terror lingering at the edge of a hollowed out existence.

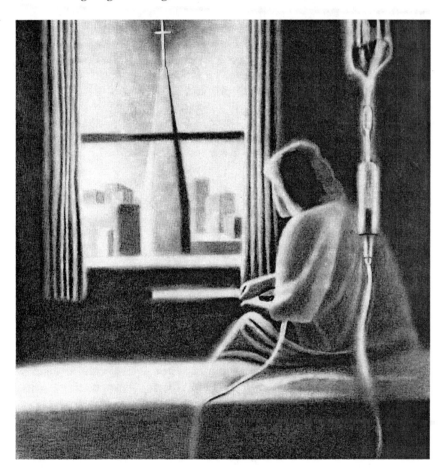

Figure 16. Robert Pope, "Steeple", 1990. Charcoal on paper, 32,4 x 32.4 cm. Courtesy of the Robert Pope Foundation, Hantsport, Nova Scotia.

The use of sketches (rather than paintings or photographs) as a way of getting near to pre-reflective moments is no accident. The indeterminacy of light and dark, the evocation of people caught in a time and setting are indicative of a state of being where clear boundaries are missing, where images rule over propositional thought. How extensive such moments are for individuals is variable, and there is no suggestion here that people do not try to reflect upon them as best they can. As already mentioned, Audre Lorde wrote that, during such times, 'Part of me flew like a big bird to the ceiling … providing a commentary (but not a coherent one)' (1980: 23). She came to the conclusion at the time that there was less to decide than to remember. Whatever she decided about speaking out about her experience, first she had to *undergo* it, to know it as a state of being in the world.

The sense that one has from Pope's pictures is that 'suffering is here' – in that place, at that time. How to conceptualise this, to give it credence beyond calling it pre-reflective? That it is important in establishing feeling is beyond question, so that what is then to be remembered, to be objectified through work of whatever kind, has been in some way *placed*, rather like the way that Frank's view from the window (re)placed his suffering.

Such moments involve a *placing of features*, something that Strawson (1959) defined as being more basic than propositional thought. Feature-placing language is of the kind, 'rain is falling or "wetness!" '. The term 'rain' in the sentence is not intended to characterise any particular referent – it is more a kind of stuff rather than being a property of a particular thing. So, it is not sensible to ask 'how many rains do you see?'. By adding criteria of identity, however, it is possible to ask, 'how many *rainstorms* do you see?' (Cussins, 1992, emphasis in the original). As Strawson argues, 'Though feature –placing sentences do not introduce particulars into our discourse, they provide a basis for this introduction.' (1959: 203). The example in our case is 'suffering is here', although the articulation of this in language inevitably involves predication – e.g. 'she is suffering'. This is because subject/predicate language involves the ascription of properties and the classification of instances through denotation. But in the recognition of 'suffering as shown' there is a consciousness *of the moment*, not of the person as a separate individual (predicate) who is denoted by the property (suffering). Feature placing involves not 'an identification of' by a third party, but 'a recognition of' a kind of moment, so that, 'Whereas the semantics of subject/predicate sentences involves *instance identification*, the semantics of feature-placing sentences involves *incidence indication*.' (Cussins, 1992: 665, emphasis in the original)

Because feature-placing does not involve a subject or a location it is not subject to truth conditions, but rather to what Cussins refers to as 'assent conditions', in which the testing of the truth/falsity of the incident is suspended. How could we judge the truth of Frank's claim about the window experience, still less that reported by Audre Lorde? In not being able to judge (or explain) these moments, we should not be tempted to exile them from our thinking about illness representation, reject them as mere romanticism, or hurry on to the finished work (painting or narrative) where the analysis of form is the preferred option.

Finished works (of illness) often contain clues as to these moments, indicating their importance. Authors ask us to entertain these assent conditions in different ways, among which is the appeal to shared givens in bodily experience. Arthur Frank appeals to this in the example of an incident (an *incidence*) in which, he said, he gave up control for wonder, when he says, 'he learned from his body'. Frank writes about a walk to the hospital for tests, knowing that he had cancer, when it began to rain heavily. As a man with cancer he had 'no aspirations to sanity', so that:

> '… wrecked as I was, when I started walking I began to feel better. I was outside and moving and really very happy. First my feet began to get wet, then my pants, and soon the water was dripping inside my jacket, but that didn't matter. Here was the world of people going to work, of puddles and grass and leaves, and I was able to be part of it.' (1991: 60)

In the course of this wetting Frank was filled with wonder at what his body could do for him, and began to appreciate it and stopped evaluating it. Here is more than 'wetness' but also, crucially, an assent by Frank to an incidence and its possible significance. There is no more that we – as readers – can say about this episode, except to accept or refuse its significance. Frank cannot make us do this; he can only endorse Wittgenstein's epithet concerning such matters: 'This is what took place here; laugh, if you can'. (Wittgenstein, 1979: 3e).

This idea of feature-placing is important not only when considering pre-reflective experience – what suffering involves – but also when we come to consider how these moments are communicated to others, mediated by works. As I have said, there can be no consideration of pre-reflective thought except through reflection. The way that this reflection constructs the moment does not, of course, mean that there is no pre-reflective experience. And while this way of speaking suggests that such moments 'come before', we shall see that this cannot only be the case. Indeed, if works of illness are to convey the significance of that experience, such moments must be made to 'come after' as well, so that the reader and viewer might also metaphorically, if not literally, shudder in turn.

Illness and the Sublime

Speaking of serious illness and its treatment in terms of horror raises new questions about its representation. In saying that horror 'makes an appearance' that does not need to be explained, I have suggested that its representation cannot be one of specification or denotation alone. The issue here is not one of distinguishing between forms of discourse (the 'seeable and the sayable'), or the semiotic (the symbolic and the indexical/iconic). Rather, we need to examine the way that the terrors of serious illness and the threat of death are re-presented in works of various kinds. That horror makes its appearance is undoubted; that it can be made to appear again – even unwittingly – is also without question. The artistic mode in which this has been achieved in modern times is the sublime (Shaw, 2006). This position has been advocated within a postmodern framework by Lyotard, who concluded from Edmund Burke's *A Philosophical Enquiry* (1757/1990) that, 'there is another kind of pleasure that is bound to a passion far stronger than satisfaction, and that is suffering and impending death' (Lyotard, 1984: 40). For Burke, ideas of pain, sickness and death 'fill the mind with horror' (1990: 36), but compared with feelings of pleasure, are more powerful. This spiritual passion is synonymous with terror, which if it is too close – imminent – produces only fear but, 'at certain distances, and with certain modifications, they may be and they are delightful, as we every day experience' (Burke, 1990: 36-37). The sublime is therefore a response rooted in terror made tolerable (indeed, 'delightful') by distance and modification.

Burke set out a further feature of the terrible, which is that its bounds cannot be discerned, so that it cannot be seen distinctly. He was adamant that obscurity was essential to a sense of the sublime, leading to the idea that its form approached infinity and therefore that it cannot be clearly represented. For this reason he was critical of attempts to paint the terrible, complaining that in all the pictures he had seen of hell he was at something of a loss to know whether the artist was attempting something ludicrous. For Burke, the way to approach the sublime was with words, through allusion, and therefore via poetry.

Burke's view that the sublime is unrepresentable (or that it cannot be conveyed clearly, which is not quite the same thing) is allied to a Romantic vision, to be found both in Romantic poetry and in paintings such as those by

Salvator Rosa (1615-73), whose canvases often depicted figures against the background of awe inspiring natural scenes. Among the 'modifications' that Rosa used was the device of showing the world with the sun setting, giving an impression of a scene to be overtaken by darkness in which the clarity of objects would give way to their formlessness. By comparison, Goya in his cabinet pictures, led the viewer closer to dangerous scenes, where, for example, a desolate landscape shows a coach having being attacked by brigands and the travellers brutally murdered. The power of these pictures lay in depicting scenes that the viewer might experience, which Goya continued in his painting *Yard with Lunatics*. In this painting the theme is not so much the blackness of the asylum yard as the blackness of lunacy itself, a dreaded condition that filled Goya's generation with nightmarish fears, just as cancer does today (Klein, 1998).

In Romantic paintings, nature's indifference provides the backdrop to the action, its allusive power the engulfment of the person in the formlessness of space dominated by the elements. Drawing again on Caillois's (1984) intriguing essay on mimicry, we might say that the darkness in these paintings is not a mere absence of light but a positivity, in which the lack of distinction between person and surroundings constitutes a permeability of boundaries, an analogue of that boundary dissipation that defines the abject state. For Caillois, the assimilation to space is contiguous with a disturbance of time, in which the assumptions about the course of the everyday are fundamentally disturbed. The viewer is drawn into the scene as into the 'lure of material space', where that virtual descent into formlessness is the instantiation of 'terror' in the picture. And yet there is a kind of delight and consolation to be found there, not least in the indifference of the scene. In her essay on being ill, Virginia Woolf overcame her yearning for words that could communicate the experience of lying ill in bed. She recognized that, lying recumbent, 'the sky is discovered to be so different [from this] that really it is a little shocking' (1994: 321). She continued in her reflection on the role of nature in illness, to say that:

> Wonderful to relate, poets have found religion in Nature; people live in the country to learn from plants. It is in their indifference that they are comforting. That snowfield of the mind, where man has not trodden, is visited by the cloud, kissed by the falling petal, as, in another sphere, it is the great artists, the Miltons, the Popes, who console, not by their thought of us, but by their forgetfulness. (1994: 322). See also Coates, (2002).

The sublime is that which is aesthetic first and, if at all beautiful (in a conventional sense), only secondarily so. Among its modern expositors was Francis Bacon, for whom pain has been described as a 'gorgeous spectacle' in his evocation of bodily existence (Cooper, 2002). He destroyed an early painting, *Wound for a Crucifixion* [1934], which is described as 'set in a hospital ward, or corridor, with the wall painted dark green to waist height and cream above, with a long, horizontal black line in between. On a sculptor's armature was a large section of human flesh: a specimen wound, and a "very beautiful wound" according to Bacon's recollection' (quoted in Harrison, 2005: 122). In spite of this, it is reported that Bacon denied that his subject was horror, and compared his paintings to those 'so grand it takes away the horror' (Harrison, 2005: 212). This is consistent with Burke's idea that delight follows from distance and modification, though in its modern form the sublime 'seizes, strikes and inflicts sensation' (Boileau, quoted in Lyotard, 1984: 39). For Lyotard, the sublime concerns absolutes – like suffering and death – that 'can only be considered without reason, [where] the imagination and the ability to present fail to provide appropriate representations' (1984: 40). It is this failure of representation that constitutes, in a negative but powerful way, the inexpressibility of suffering and the horror that may accompany it.

What is it that is so terrifying? According to Lyotard it is that the ongoingness (the 'happenings') of life will no longer continue to happen. Such happenings are part and parcel of the narrative flow of one's life, the idea (a luxury for those diagnosed with serious disease) that life is a story, with a timeline that is extendable, reaching out into the future. Art, and aesthetic conduct in general, distances this terror, producing a kind of 'delight'. Thanks to this, 'the soul is returned to the agitated zone between life and death, and this agitation is its health and its life' (Lyotard, 1984: 40). This effect cannot be achieved (as Burke insisted) through depiction but must test its limits through surprise, through shocking combinations. It is this that says something along the lines of, 'This is happening, and it is happening here, now'. It witnesses indeterminacy by partaking of it, establishing in the aesthetic of the sublime an affirmative presence, not the failed attempt to represent an ethereal world. This is not an occasion for mourning but the celebration of an emancipatory potential (Rampley, 2000: 237), something similar to Foucault's (1980) idea of 'problematising life as a work of freedom'. The horrors of serious illness and death may be beyond our understanding but they are not beyond our reach.

This idea of the sublime as an instantiation of the unknown sets up a different view of the horror of serious illness from that which would position it as quite outside representation. It is outside specification, to be sure, but can be made to re-appear through distancing and modification, in effect through ascetic practice. What needs to be underlined here is that the horror of illness infects the mundane, presents itself with ordinary events that so often emphasise its powers to engulf. It survives in these fragmented events and in the 'crush of thoughts that do not get out because they all try to push forward and are wedged in the door' (Wittgenstein, 1979: 3e). These events and thoughts form the aesthetic basis for representation because they are of the present; they are sensuously here, now. This idea of the transmutation of suffering by virtue of our being embodied is reminiscent of the view put forward by Walter Benjamin:

> If the theory is correct that feeling is not located in the head, that we sentiently experience a window, a cloud, a tree, not in our brains but, rather, in the place where we see it, then we are, in looking at our beloved, too, outside ourselves. But in a torment of tension and ravishment. Our feeling, dazzled, flutters like a flock of birds in the woman's radiance. And as birds seek refuge in the leafy recesses of a tree, feelings escape into the shaded wrinkles, the awkward movements and inconspicuous blemishes of the body we love, where they can lie low in safety. And no passer-by would guess that it is just here, in what is defective and censurable, that the fleeting darts of adoration nestle. (1986: 68)

This excerpt can be read as a further example of the way that the sublime is grasped in the sensual, and that bearing witness to it is effectively made in the context of the transmutation of what is deemed abhorrent. It is consistent with the idea that the sublime, in the context of illness representation in the modern world, deals with what is happening in the here and now, that a life lived as an affirmative presence is not one removed to an ethereal plane, which would be a simple reversal of the 'edgelessness' of abjection. Instead, one might take as illustrative of the alternative position the ethical view espoused by Gillian Rose. As a way of remaining in the sphere of the sensuous, close to what she calls the 'edges of life', she adopted the recommendation to 'Keep your mind in hell and despair not'. (1995: 98).

I read this as: keeping one's mind in hell is not a capitulation to abjection, but a precondition for its transmutation. This reading is consistent with the idea that the sublime be conceived of as 'an offering or gesture that takes place at the limit of art' (Shaw, 2006: 150), so that there is an acknowledgement of the contradiction that the apparent emptiness of illness can give life a different sort of meaning. We need now to examine exactly how pictures and stories do their work to make this possible, and with this to return finally to the role of the aesthetic in depicting the world of the ill person.

Chapter 6

Works and Worlds

While it would be mistaken to think that one can talk about works of illness *outside* of social developments, it is not so to think about them *beside* their historical context. This is to shift away from a steady focus upon social context as something that turns representations into instances of production or consumption, so describing how they came into being, how they were disseminated, to whom and with what effects on others and their creators. If, on the other hand, one wishes to address the question of *the work done* by stories, paintings and photographs about illness, then attention must be re-directed. Only by allowing ourselves to be taken aside by them, or to see how others are taken aside, can we also entertain them beside social context. Without being willing to do this, issues concerning the problematisation of the situation of the seriously ill and how this is to be understood remain opaque. Or rather, they are thrown back into the everyday world of the sufferer, and remain immune to the ideas and practices of institutional forms of knowledge. Their potential as configured solutions to ways of living in the world passes by the specialist. This matters because the current circumstances that call out to ill people to communicate their situation are differently readable through those individual efforts. Perhaps one should not say differently readable but differently apprehensible, so making works informative of the way that, in today's world, basic issues about illness are met and understood by sick and healthy in their turn.

I want to relate the arguments made so far to some recent developments in health care. One concerns the differentiation of control as medicine makes individuals responsible for monitoring (before) and maintaining (after) episodes of illness. This removes the patient from the environs of the clinic as a definitive feature of their relationship to medicine. (This relationship continues, but it is no longer the same, as patients consulting their doctor with a print out from Internet websites can tell us.) The second is the move to make experiences of illness – often involving treatment and its consequences – public and sharable. Taken together, and put alongside the grooming of the patient as consumer, these changes create a situation in which illness escapes (though not entirely) the bounds of medicine. The world of the 'whole patient' – or even the complete sufferer, a term of uncertain application – is gradually being supplanted by a condition in which individuals are differentiated by the analytic procedures of medicine. In a complementary and yet unavoidable way, for individuals to pass through this system in which their bodies are fragmented and objectified means that their biographical subjectivity is *diffracted*, sometimes even before it is disrupted by the onset of serious disease. This concerns not only medical technology in its material aspect but also the moral and legal consequences of being monitored or maintained in our social lives.

The way we might think of this is that the 'patient in context' is being dislodged or de-positioned, so as to produce the conditions for both social criticism and critical reflection. In the case of people with AIDS, for example, social criticism appears as stigma, while critical reflection is encouraged by social movements concerned with changing attitudes toward sexuality. It would seem that the major social health movements around AIDS and breast cancer in the 1990s borrowed techniques and ideologies from the emancipatory movements regarding class, sexuality and women's rights. In that context, the works made by people like Jo Spence and the American artist/photographer Hannah Wilke, for example, can be seen as being different from those (such as the work of Arthur Frank or Martha Hall) that resist the technological usurpation of care. However, in both cases, the pictures and stories created served to make public what was formerly a private experience (between the patient and his or her doctor) and also to criticise the medical and social situation of individuals who are ill.

The question then becomes, how do stories and paintings direct viewers and readers to the fact that they are doing this kind of work? Is it not enough that they deal with relevant content, are in some cases considered artworks (of a kind), and that they produce some effects upon the reader or viewer? The answer to this must be qualified, if only because the way that these matters are related (they are not features that act quite separately) concerns the relationship of the work to the grounds from which it is drawn and the audience to which it speaks. These are matters of exemplification, possession and framing.

Picturing and Possession: how works of illness exemplify

At this point we need to address directly the question of how works that deal with serious illness convey meaning; or rather, how they tell about illness as an aesthetic condition. The latter is of course a more specific issue, for there will be meanings other than the aesthetic to be read into or out of an essay or painting. Illness narratives are more usually examined for their content about the illness experience or for their way of reconstructing the biography of the persons concerned. In the matter of how works – in narrative or paintings – 'picture' illness, the issue links both to the way that works signify and to the way in which they come to be regarded potentially as art. This issue of how artworks claim to be just that – works – was summarised by Susan Sontag in her critique of the role of interpretation, when she said (about any work of art) that 'the function of criticism should be to show *how it is what it is*, even *that it is what it is*, rather than to show what *it means*' (Sontag, 1978: 14, emphasis in original). This phrase captures the idea that how works signify is bound up with how they appear ontologically, to be a certain kind of object. We are familiar with this in the general context of poems and paintings that not only say something but also, in how they do it, are held to be particular kinds of artefacts. In relation to the particular issue of essays, poems, paintings, or photographs concerning illness, the question arises as to what it is that must be shown if such works are to be seen to be what they are. In order to discuss this issue I shall use the term 'picturing' to cover both how paintings exemplify and how narratives describe in order to express as well as denote feeling.

The answer to this question is that works of illness must exemplify – indeed express – suffering so as to engage the reader/viewer with the horrors faced, whether or not these horrors were or cannot be overcome. The aesthetic in these cases is not the idea of a beautiful object, but an evocation of the sublime, where this means the creation of a 'screen' through which the gaze of the terrors of illness can be contemplated. The key issue here is that these terrors are what people with serious illness have to suffer, if not to face, so that no story of treatment and recovery, of remission or its failure, can be grounded except by acknowledging horror in some form. The creation of a work – as a screen – involves a transmutation of horror in the act of realising its aesthetic figuration. The double point here is that this transmutation necessitates a display in which the terrors are symbolically set forth, and that the way that this is done announces the artefact as a 'work in itself'.

The significance of works of illness depends upon *them* presenting (or re-presenting) illness in terms of an aesthetic, and that this aesthetic lies in the evocation of a figurative world. Works transform their authors and other people's understanding of the world through displays that both create a sense of the present and articulate significant features of social life. Catching up the threads of the moment to create the possibility of another way of living alludes to a totality, a way of being, while at the same time lending significance to specific things said or done. In terms of illness experience, this means that the illness account or the picture witnesses experience through the evocation of a world that is figuratively, as well as literally real. If the account were not of this kind – if it were 'only' a story that recounted events, or a photograph that 'merely' showed that this happened then, or that the patient was told these things – the reader/viewer would neither be repelled nor moved by the representation of how illness is borne.

This approach implies a treatment of the way that pictures and stories mediate experience, or to put it more forcefully, that these works are given qualities or powers that enable the reader or viewer to make again something that the work not only denotes but exemplifies. I have already moved away from the idea that illness narratives are transparent windows into a person's experience, or that they tell us the story of that person's life. Instead, these stories and pictures are better thought of as 'replicative machines' that allow something important to be made again, to be seen anew by others, to be grasped afresh. This means that they share with art objects the characteristic of being made up, and the world that they help to configure is a made up world. This does not mean that this world is illusory but that the *elusory* qualities concerning suffering and mortality can be in some way grasped if not named through circumscription.

In her treatise on pain, Scarry made the concept of *work* central in her proposal that pain (and by extension, suffering) is an intentional state without an intentional object. About the work of objectifying pain, she said:

> The more it realizes itself in its object, the closer it is to the imagination, to art, to culture; the most it is unable to bring forth an object or, bringing it forth, is then cut off from its object, the more it approaches the condition of pain. (Scarry, 1985: 169).

Scarry's argument is that pain is to be understood through its realization in forms that, in being graspable by others, make this a social rather than a private state, or in her terms, the self-contained loop within the body becomes an 'equivalent' loop now projected into the external world. The nature of this equivalence is, of course, not obvious, and provides the ground for much of the analysis in this chapter. The change that is undergone in the transformation effected by the creation of the artefact follows from the move away from 'the wholly passive and acute suffering of physical pain' to the 'self-regulated and modest suffering of work'. Work, in this as in other contexts, denotes both an activity and a product. As for the activity, this is not merely a re-assemblage of things but an act that issues in something that conveys an idea, by projecting an imaginary order; it is, in that sense, world-making. In terms of work as a product, these objects are in Scarry's terms 'fragments of world alteration' (1985: 171). In an important way, works of any kind are sharable but are also crucially constructive. As she concludes:

> The advantage of material culture over a culture of belief is …difficult to overstate. In work, then, pain is moderated into sustained discomfort; and the objects of imagining, though individually moderated into fragmentary artefacts, are collectively translated into the structures of civilization that have nothing modest about them. (Scarry, 1985: 172).

Redirecting attention towards aesthetic activity 'as work' allows an investigation of the way that texts or pictures are made up. In turn, this allows a discussion of how these works make something available to others, either fellow sufferers or the healthy. Taking this line of argument, detailed attention to 'works of illness as fragments of world alteration' offers new insights into how ideas of illness and practices relating to it are organised.

To make use of examples is easiest, perhaps, by reference to paintings; all of Robert Pope's drawings and paintings would fit this description. But so would some famous novels (with which we are not dealing here), as well as a number of essays (illness narratives) that convey 'what it is like' to be seriously ill. I would consider Gillian Rose's *Love's Work*, Anatole Broyard's *Intoxicated By My Illness* and Arthur Frank's *At the Will of the Body* to be in this realm. In a phrase, the other side of the 'work in itself' is the person's 'world of illness' into which the reader/viewer is ushered by the text and the line.

Showing how serious illness appeared, what it did to one's life, how one responded to its claims, is an aesthetic enterprise when this showing exemplifies the significant character of suffering. The idea of exemplification is more than a telling, because it is crucially also a showing, and one that involves displaying what cannot be named directly. As I have argued, horror, suffering and love are evoked or expressed in these works, and it is this mode of articulation that makes them what they are.

In order to explain this, I shall find it useful to move between picturing and textual description, as these are so often used in everyday life as metaphors for one another. Robert Pope's paintings were discussed earlier in terms of the way that he evokes features of key moments in terms of shading of both people and setting together. This metaphorical expression of mood is also present in Gillian Rose's book, in which she paints a similarly dark picture of the place where she must wait to receive her chemotherapy treatment, in a hospital in Birmingham:

> In the amorphous reception area of the hospital, large oblong notices in five oriental languages are perched above the lintels of the lifts to the right of the main entrance of the hospital and over the entrance to the main interior corridor, the longest corridor in Europe. The English version declares; 'If you feel you have waited an unduly long time, please contact the ambulance clerk or the receptionist.' The people milling here cover the spectrum of the life-cycle: they look like 'Musselmen', the working prisoners of labour and death camps who give up the will to live, and lose the fierce, burning glare of starvation in their eyes. Hordes of people sitting in rows are condemned by those notices to the indifference marked by their contrary signification. All access and egress lies through this dispiriting terrace of deprivation. (Rose, 1995: 81).

This descriptive passage evokes, like Pope's paintings, a similar sense of illness involving waiting, except in this case it is coloured by borrowing properties associated with people 'condemned' in camps, while at the same time pointing directly to the 'contrary signification' conveyed by the notices on the wall. At this point I do not want to consider differences between text and picture, but would draw attention to the way in which both so often appear together – are made together – in everyday life. Both this descriptive excerpt and some of Pope's drawings in the hospital evoke that sense of illness as desolation. But, the question needs to be asked, are they 'desolate' works?

To help us here we can refer to Goodman's (1968) distinction between exemplification and denotation in representation. To *denote* is to use a label to refer to something, so that a picture may denote a hospital ward. However, some of Robert Pope's drawings may be said to be 'dark' pictures, in which case they also *exemplify* or show forth the property of darkness. In this sense, the pictures do not denote the colour 'black' but are instead denoted by the predicate 'black'. That is, they both possess this quality and refer to it. Merely to have a quality (such as being a 'heavy hammer') is not to exemplify weightiness. Exemplification is possession *plus reference*, and the form of this reference is for the vehicle to allow itself to be referred to by the predicate. Goodman's regular illustration for this is the tailor's swatch, which exemplifies certain properties of the textile, made possible by its being cut out from the world of clothing, so that it becomes a framed, miniature exemplar of that material. Its references here are literal, in that if one chooses the cloth based upon the swatch one will purchase a textile with that colour, that weave, that finish. (One will not, however, purchase a garment composed of lots of swatches stitched together. The issue of which properties are exemplified is clearly important, and one that we need to return to when discussing the way that works are understood.)

The term 'dark' as a descriptive quality of Pope's pictures can be taken literally, so that some of his paintings and drawings may be said to exemplify blackness as a property. But they do more than this. Several of Pope's pictures also express a sense of desolation and despair, features that might or might not have been felt by Pope himself at the time. This evocation is made possible by the borrowing from other realms of what blackness might imply, as well as drawing the figures concerned in such a way as to denote their passive relationship to the hospital setting. This borrowing from other realms is the necessary condition for *expression*, as Goodman defines it, which is a mode of symbolization involving figurative possession, the exemplification of borrowed qualities. So, Pope's pictures are not 'desolate' in the same way that they are 'black', because the latter property is possessed in a literal not a metaphorical sense. Only when we bring these two terms together under the word 'dark' do we allude to the joint condition in which pictures show forth both literally and metaphorically possessed features. These are then 'patterns and properties that reorganize experience, relating actions not usually associated or distinguishing others not usually differentiated, thus enriching allusion or sharpening discrimination' (Goodman, 1968: 65).

This distinction between literal and metaphorical possession is important because it allows for the fact that a picture or poem need not express what it denotes (delineates, says) or denote what it expresses. In the case of the drawings by Robert Pope that we have been considering, the 'darkness' of the pictures serves to underline the conjunction between these conditions, but it does not determine it. So, to describe experiences of suffering is not necessarily to express them, while suffering can be evoked through depictions that are not of suffering as such. This allows for the important difference between accounts of illness that set out (denote) a story of symptoms, treatment and recovery and those that do this but also express the condition of affliction. The former have all the features of narrative plots – they are accounts of events – but do not express the suffering involved; the latter evoke a world in which the sufferer lives, because expressive symbolization is of the work itself. Going back to Scarry's proposal that an artefact is 'a fragment of world alteration' we can see now that this is not a matter of changing the world literally. It is rather a matter of such works (of art, of illness) *proposing a figurative world* – a world of illness – into which the reader or viewer is invited.

Consider again the self-portrait by Elissa Hugens Aleshire (see Figure 7, p.89), who painted this picture some time after her operation for the removal of a breast, following the diagnosis of cancer. The picture is drawn from the collection *Art.Rage.Us.* published by the *Breast Cancer Fund of America* (1998). It shows four images of her, three partial figures and one, centre-front, a complete figure. It is this figure that commands attention as it shows her naked to the waist, the scar of her missing right breast alongside the 'healthy' left breast. She looks straight ahead, into the mirror that (she tells us) she used in order to create the painting. It is an open look, what she terms in the accompanying comment 'the first real look at myself after surgery'. To the side and behind this central figure are three others. They are partly hidden, and in each case hide the missing breast. To the viewer's left she is shown wearing a blouse. To the right, and behind, we see only her face and a bare shoulder, her chest obscured by the two images in front. She holds her fingers to her chin, giving the impression of a quizzical attitude. The fourth figure, to the viewer's right, is only half in the picture, holding up her hand to cover the site of the missing right breast. By this device we are shown three part-figures whose anatomical completeness is preserved (by obscuration), and one whole figure who reveals that she is anatomically incomplete. The total picture works to suggest the achievement of self-recognition against the background of fear of revelation. In the course of this portrayal, the mastectomy scar so clearly depicted is given a different context. It is re-figured along with the artist as sufferer. This does not mean that its original (one might say, ab-original) power to evoke horror is entirely removed. (That this is not so can be demonstrated by showing the picture afresh to different viewers).

Rather, the suffering that is indicated by the wound is given form, re-contextualising the scar and giving it new meaning. The picture was not created by attempting to displace attention from the scar, but rather by facing it and re-figuring it. As Elissa Aleshire comments:

> A week before the surgery, I had drawn a 'before' picture, and I promised myself I would do an 'after'. It took about three months to work up to it. This painting was the first real look at myself after my surgery, and at first I was embarrassed to even show anyone. But in fact, the process healed me, sitting in front of a mirror looking at an image that scared me. (Breast Cancer Fund, 1998: 101)

This comment shows the act of painting to involve confrontation with the mastectomy scar in order that it might be transformed. In order to look beyond the scar, she had first to look *at* it. This indicates that horror is not dismissed in the course of such portrayals but that its powers are diminished in the course of being given a form, a shape. However, painting is not an objectification of horror as such (for then it could not 'heal') but the projection of the artist's recovery of herself from the grip of illness and its terrors. What the image achieves – using multiple figures – is a sense of coherence for Elissa Aleshire through an expressive portrayal of that recovery. The picture is an exemplification of her position – it stands forth as an open acknowledgement and acceptance of what is – while also being an expression (in Goodman's terms) of qualities that are elusive to specification. The idea of metaphorical possession refers here to the figurative projection of a world (of illness) of which the image stands as if a fragment. As a fragment of such a figurative world (which in its assemblage of feelings is as actual as any literal depiction), the image is bounded by a space-time of experience (looking at the picture, painting the picture) that sets it off from the mundane world. This does not imply a separation from the world of disease and surgery, but the fabrication of a way of being in relation to things, so that they are imbued with meanings that previously did not belong to them.

While the imaged world of recovery (of illness-as borne) is a fabricated one, dealing in metaphors, it is not an ethereal one, in the sense of being wholly transcendent. It is fabricated by means of paint, and by virtue of remaining engaged with the mundane world that our bodies occupy. No transformation of suffering could be achieved by a portrayal that had wholly lost touch with the possibility of pain. To portray a 'world of suffering as borne' it is necessary that the picture remains an exemplar of pain, that it continues to show forth those features (e.g. the mastectomy scar) in the course of expressing the self-possession referred to above. This should not be thought of as the projection of any 'self' at all, but is an aesthetic judgement based upon the fact that the painting (as of Elissa Aleshire) does two things. It invites a restoration of coherence, and expresses feelings that were previously inchoate. As experiences, they are to be sought both in the act of painting (which 'heals') and in the contemplation of the image by the viewer. Inasmuch as it is seen as coherent, the picture is comprehended as a totality, and as such a fragment of the world to which it refers, (i.e. it is a sample of 'illness-as-borne'). The image thus stands both in the mundane world (of paint, of media, of spaces of observation) and in the figurative world that it fabricates. And because the fabrication of this world requires work on the part of the artist, and the contemplative effort on the part of the viewer, its expressive potential is realised as the achievement of distance from horror and pain. That distance – which is common to all ascetic practice – is created by the objectifying skills of the artist, through which pain and horror are given communicative form. It is in the act of *making* that the picture of 'suffering-as-borne' is given shape and form.

Written accounts of illness can also express as well as exemplify, and exemplify as well as denote. The degree to which they do this will depend upon the way in which the author uses metaphor to draw upon different realms in order to evoke something that cannot be literally seen, cannot be adequately circumscribed. When Anatole Broyard says, 'What goes through your mind when you're lying full of nuclear dye, under a huge machine that scans all your bones for evidence of treason?' (1992: 22), he invites the reader to contemplate illness not merely as if it were treachery, but, in the context of the work, to see the world with the eyes he fashions. This is rather different – and importantly different – from saying that he asks us to 'see the world through his eyes'. First, there is not a single ('the') world to be seen. Second, we do not see *through* Broyard's eyes – organs forming part of his body, taken literally. Instead, we see *with* (not through) eyes that are fashioned metaphorically in the image Broyard creates for us. This is an extension of the point made earlier that we contemplate 'with the eyes of horror'. The wordsmith and the painter fashion their works so as to give them powers of fascination, elision and allusion. More concretely, it has been proposed that, in some cultures, stone images are not just specified (refined) but also empowered by the addition of recognizable elements. 'A stone standing for a person is given 'eyes', not so that the stone will resemble the person in question but rather so that the stone will possess powers of sight as its counterpart did.' (Summers, 1991a: 253).

To underline a point made earlier, all of these works invite the viewer/reader not just to see differently, or even to see like another, but to *see as* a participant in a figured world. In consequence, we do not turn away so readily from horror given a new guise, one that forms a screen in the face of which we are (to use Lacan's phrase) invited to lay down the weapons of our gaze. Works of illness – as with all artworks – hold our attention within a space that is figured by the artefact, in which the space that emerges between the literal and the metaphoric parallels the agitated zone between life and death, which Burke and Lyotard proposed to be 'the life of the soul'.

In sum, depictions of illness do more than denote, for example, 'cancer' or exemplify 'being a cancer patient'. The aesthetic mode crucially involves the transmutation of horrors, offering up what is held unspeakable (or unseeable) in a figurative display that conveys the symbolic meaning of illness. This kind of portrayal is central to all endeavours that evoke a world that is figuratively real, so that what is expressed is a sensibility (an idea) rather than an inchoate feeling. To grasp this idea involves an act of imagination, one that transcends the immediacy of response that constitutes the mundane world. These portrayals draw the viewer closer to the significant object (on the one hand, the desired body, on the other, the abhorrent body). It is this engagement with the elements of horror and desire that enables the aesthetic project to surpass the responses of pity or indignation. To analyse this further we need to examine the idea of world-making in more detail, and what this could mean for realising illness as a work of freedom.

The Limits of the Visual

While what can be seen – can be denoted – is important, this must not be confused with what works of illness express. Indeed, the self-portrait by Elissa Aleshire and the photograph of Stefan Wahrlich have in common the fact that they 'show' what is not there. In one case it is a woman's missing breast, in the other case a man's missing leg. It has been said already that the mere revelation of a scar, of a site of amputation, is not synonymous with the portrayal of suffering. If anything, pictures of wounds are more likely to elicit fear and loathing. Making visible is clearly not the same as making meaning. However, the issue of visibility is an issue for the chronically ill in their day-to-day appearances in public. To be visibly impaired, or to live under the threat of stigma, requires using procedures to avoid being discredited in the eyes of others. These procedures vary according to the degree to which one's illness is visible, so that where it can be 'covered up' one's physical failing can be hidden. In the general case of the images selected for discussion here, prostheses are available for women who have received mastectomies, and for people who have had a leg amputated.

These ways of covering up serve as methods of normalization that allow the person concerned to pass unnoticed among the healthy and the able-bodied. What this avoids for the majority is the social embarrassment associated with a sense of mortal decline, particularly in contexts affirmative of health, beauty and pleasure. Such alignments with social schedules (schedules for how to appear physically adept, how to walk – the most basic requirements of social involvement) are necessary displays of consonance with general qualities of the group. While these qualities will be given form in a variety of ways and different contexts (the social conventions of stylistic behaviours) certain key elements are conserved in the requirement that they be identified as 'this' or 'that' style.

Where, however, a person is unable to conceal the marks of illness, they may be forced to do other work (often narrative work) in order to legitimise their claim to be just 'an ordinary person'. That is, the visibility of difference calls for explanation that can keep at bay the summary response of exclusion following a sense of 'horror' at what has been revealed. In this case, too, the afflicted person seeks a stability of identity through a kind of resistance. This resistance is to the change in group-qualities that are transformed through the person's inability to display their required form (i.e. through an inability to appear complete, or to walk with ease and grace).

Issues of stigma primarily involve the visual because they are matters of alignment with social schedules (Goffman, 1976). As such, displays of behaviour that contribute attempts at normalization are quite different in their mode of signification from the portraits of 'suffering-as-borne' that were described above. This is not because, on the one hand, suffering is hidden and, on the other, it is shown. This is altogether too simple. It is because in the one case what is being preserved (through display and exemplification) are the attributes or qualities definitive of a particular group of persons, and of its outlook. The stability of such qualities (the maintenance of social identity) is the paramount goal here, whether the stigmata can be hidden or whether they have to be legitimated and contextualised because they cannot be hidden. In this case, the locus of meaning is 'on the body', so that consonance and difference are both read directly from what may be seen in the disfigurement or in the pronounced limp. These readings are conventionalised, and because the schedules of normality and difference are those in which we are well schooled, give rise to immediate perceptions on this dimension. The point is that both afflicted and observers may point to the part of the body that is 'offensive to the eye'. We need look no further.

Such is not the case with portrayals of 'suffering-as-borne'. The figurative portrayal of an illness world is of something that cannot be isolated on the canvas or print because it is not there to be seen. The portrayal of 'persons' rather than 'objects' involves a re-designation of the viewer as someone receiving the message or the picture anew. This fashioning of the other's illness world 'within' the observer constitutes the re-figuration of him/her with respect to the mundane world of pain and suffering. This re-figuring is coterminous with understanding, and shows that signification in this case is not to do with communicating meaning about objects, but is all about the instantiation of persons. And, we should add, about the instantiation of worlds that they have made.

If we re-affirm the need for suffering to be given expressive form, and for the work of fabrication and contemplation to be seen as constructive practices, then portrayals must exist at one time in both the mundane and the sublime (the obverse of suffering). These two spheres are irreducible to each other. To try to *see* the sublime in the visually rendered medium is to reify visuality into a replica of the world in its mundane aspect. This is precisely what portrayals of suffering (as with all art) do not do, in their attempt to surpass the passivity of suffering in order to witness the person's response to it.

The stress upon the visual in the analysis of such pictures is partly a consequence of the attempt to 'distinguish the visual from the verbal', perhaps in the cause of dislodging linguistic imperialism (for a critique see Mitchell, 1994; Summers, 1991b). However, by accentuating the difference between presentational and discursive forms in this way, the conceptual work of portrayal is degraded in the analysis as a consequence of the conflation of words and ideas. As Adorno (1984) makes clear, the attempt to focus on the visual tends towards specification of what pictures represent. And yet, the meaning of portraits (as works of art) is to be realised in what he called their 'rational control .... over all that is heterogeneous to them' (1984; 141). The portrayal of suffering does not only find meaning but retains it through its re-construction of the sensuous experiences of those who contemplate the image. In brief, because portrayal expresses suffering and the world of the ill person, it exemplifies something about life and how it can be lived. That is why these pictures are more than ways of seeing (bodies); as already concluded, they are ways of 'seeing-as' (figurative persons). This argument points to these pictures' power to be *context-making* rather than merely being context determined. In turn, this is the source and the continued meaning of what they show forth, so that portrayals of suffering are – as with all art – 'a vision of the non-visual' (Adorno, 1984: 142).

All this goes to show that picturing suffering is more than a matter of visual depiction, more than resemblance and revelation. What is at issue is the possibility of the observer sustaining a look, a look that is not overwhelmed by the stare of the object portrayed. This stare is the power of the image to overwhelm, to suffuse the observer with pity, horror or revulsion. How the look of the observer might be sustained is a question of *re-presenting* the suffering of the ill person, allowing pain to be given expressive form and thereby enabling the observer to reciprocate in the establishment of a compassionate understanding of the sick. Even then, nothing can be guaranteed about how people will view images or even read accounts of serious illness.

Portrayals of illness – pictures or written accounts – are, in their different ways, precisely like this because of the context in which suffering is muted in the cause of medical treatment. It is this anaesthesia consequent upon diagnosis and treatment that is overcome by the presentational work of the painting, account or photograph, works that have the power to restore coherence and potential to the person concerned. We might go further and repeat that such works not only restore feeling but also sustain the capacity to feel, and this potential is there not only for the artist but also for others who read and look. The display that is figuratively set out in the painting or photograph makes communicable and subject to discourse the relationships between illness and the social world. What apparently began as art (or like art) can then become the stuff of ideology and the politics of care.

Real and Actual Worlds

When discussing the effects of illness in Chapter 5 I began by saying that, with the shock of diagnosis, the person's world is often drained of lightness, something that accompanies a fall into the mundane. This proposal rests upon an assumption that people live not in one 'real world', but in worlds actualised through conjecture, fantasy and material culture. The sphere of art is one in which, like that of the media, people can figure themselves in different ways, imagine the possibilities that life might offer them and also make – in the sense of fabricate – the material settings in which these ideas can best be sustained. It is this capacity, and with that the worlds that it makes possible, that is in danger of being displaced with the onset of serious illness. Metaphorical expression is no less actual than matters that are taken literally, though it can often be designated as 'less real'. Whatever the case, works of illness, as artefacts, are fragments that partake of literal worlds, of the mundane; and do so in the course of being lent properties that they come, metaphorically and actually, to possess.

The view that the aesthetic sphere is essentially distinct comes traditionally from the belief that art is separate from the everyday world, a view that was held by Simmel (1959a) and is still held today (Lyotard, 1984). Illness accounts, in bearing witness to horrors and revelations, partake of both the mundane and the sublime, which are apprehended as such only in relation to each other, and which are irreducible one to the other. But the sublime is always apprehended by virtue of the mundane, in the sensuous grounding of the body in the world (Merleau-Ponty, 1968). Arthur Frank's window experience partook of both mundane and aesthetic worlds, which location defines it as a fragment in relation to the totalities of meaning that it expresses. This situation can be elucidated by recourse to Simmel's (1959a) illustration of a painting of a vase, which he uses as an example of how certain artefacts stand in two worlds at one and the same time. More precisely, Simmel pointed to the handle (on the vase) as that point where these two worlds are both located. The handle is both the means by which the vase is grasped and is aesthetically pleasing, in part because its shape harmonises these two worlds. This underlines the experience of the sublime as being at once transcendent and immanent in the object, so that which is expressed in the account of illness is evoked by virtue of what happens to the person as an embodied being.

If illness accounts are a recovery of the sick person's sense of identity, having an ethical as well as an aesthetic dimension to them, then the 'handles' that provide for the articulation of the sublime will sometimes be fortuitous fragments, not always major events. In the mundane world, these are likely to concern the effects of clinical diagnosis of serious disease, of medical treatment and of the impact of events upon the family and friends. The fragment that exemplifies the sublime is not necessarily the beautiful or something that has been prejudged as significant. For example, Arthur Frank described his three months of chemotherapy as a time when 'a foot of tubing was hanging out of my chest' in order that the drugs could be delivered and blood samples taken. This line he saw as 'another flag planted by the medical system' on his body, something which he resented as much as he needed it.

> I needed the line not only for relief from pain, but also as a way of displacing my larger fears about cancer. I was able to refocus these fears – whether chemotherapy was working, how long it would go on – onto the daily problems of managing the line. (Frank, 1991: 77)

Here Frank identifies the line as something that connected him (literally) to the system that allowed fears to flourish, and yet as something that (both metaphorically and literally) provided scope for self-care. But there was more to this, in that, because the line and its exit site needed daily attention:

> The line also refocused the relationship Cathie [his wife] and I had fallen into. By the time it was installed, the hospital had pretty well taken me over. Although Cathie was usually with me during physician's visits, the doctors and nurses never acknowledged her presence (pp 77-78). ... However, Cathie took over the disinfecting, flushing and bandaging, and these tasks became a daily ritual between us. We laughed that it was our special time together, but these moments of quiet in a hectic life were a gift.... When I went back to being an inpatient, Cathie and I joked about how much better her antiseptic procedures were than those of the nurses who dressed the line (Frank, 1991: 78).

This incidence shows how a part of the world dominated by medicine (i.e. the line) signified the terrors that illness can hold, and how this was apparently transformed into a fragment that exemplified another world, one that Frank shared with his wife. This other world is a 'world of illness', in that it creates its own time-space that both of them could occupy. In the terms of the argument put forward here, this is an aesthetic achievement, a conjoint witnessing of the sublime. But it is not an achievement of other-worldliness, of an a-corporeal, a-sensual existence. The line was more than a connection between Frank and his medical carers, more than a link between him and his wife: it stood in both the realm of medicine and the 'world of illness' which the Franks were able to conjure. The sensual, in this case, was grounded in the cleaning and disinfecting of the body, by virtue of which it was possible to instantiate, to conjure this different world. The line existed simultaneously in the mundane and in the aesthetic worlds, so that on reflection it could be said to stand for something, or to signify in a different way.

What this confirms is that the production of the aesthetic sphere – creating a world of illness that is not just a world of medical care – occurs by virtue of some specific aspect of the mundane that exemplifies properties that it does not usually possess. And because what is evoked is more extensive than a single state of being, the transmutation of horror does not have to be achieved separately for each incident alone. The occasion of the line reported by Frank produces a total world – albeit brief – that has the potential to colour all of his experiences within and outside that specific world, the one of medical care.

It was not just Frank's line that existed in two worlds – as it were – but also Frank as a person, not to mention his wife. In fact, this is not to know two *separate* worlds but to live in one where, *in vivo,* the investiture of the ordinary by metaphor creates a distance that is the space of ascetic practice and enjoyment of the sublime. It is to live with horror transformed, to have created a screen through which the world and oneself is re-invested with pleasures and powers, no matter how small. To contemplate this act later – or to create an artefact that expresses this relation – is to recover that ascetic distance once more, to reconfigure one's world further in its light. To speak of it as an act of self-possession, as in relation to painting, is to confirm that way of being as 'metaphorically actual' possession.

The usefulness of speaking of acts (such as cleaning a line) alongside paintings of mastectomy scars, theatrical choreography and photographs of surgical outcome is that it underlines the way in which exemplification is a showing forth, a display, a dramatic performance. Expressive forms require that properties established as literal qualities are dislodged, somehow undone, so that other qualities may be employed from other realms. In his analysis of the Balinese cockfight, Clifford Geertz made a similar point in the following way:

> As any art form – for that finally, is what we are dealing with – the cockfight renders ordinary, everyday experience comprehensible by presenting it in terms of acts and objects which have had their practical consequences removed and been reduced (or, if you prefer, raised) to the level of sheer appearances, where their meaning can be more powerfully articulated and more exactly perceived.... An image, fiction, a model, a metaphor, the cockfight is a means of expression; its function is neither to assuage social passions nor to heighten them (though, in its play-with-fire way, it does a bit of both), but, in a medium of feathers, blood, crowds, and money, to display them. (1972: 23)

One reason for presenting this excerpt is that Geertz says that the cockfight is 'really real' only to the cocks, by which he means that the cockfight does not change the players' status in society. Put simply, the parallel to this is that works of illness do not cure disease. Whatever redemptive effects they have are realised within a configured space and time that can have – as actual effects – the relief of suffering and its communication to others. And these are no small things in a situation of fear, anxiety and isolation. When Geertz says that 'any expressive form lives in its own present – the one it itself creates' (1972: 24), he alludes to the way in which paintings and accounts establish worlds, and with that their identity as works 'in themselves'.

197

A world configured is rather like a world torn from the ordinariness of life, whose function is not to be separate (a form of escapism) but, like Simmel's (1959b) concept of 'the adventure', to re-invest life with feeling. Seen in this way, the adventure is hardly the way that most people with serious disease would describe their situation. And yet many individuals in this situation do review their lives, or re-cast their sense of existence when faced by the prospect of death. Writing about life with prostate cancer, Anatole Broyard said:

> Illness is primarily a drama, and it should be possible to enjoy it as well as to suffer it. I can see now why the Romantics were so fond of illness – the sick man sees everything as metaphor. In this phase I'm infatuated with my cancer. It stinks of revelation. (1992: 7).

For Simmel, the adventure was encouraged by 'religious moods', which on reflection, might be re-cast as experiences arising from the prospect of an earlier than expected death:

> When our earthly career strikes us as a mere preliminary phase in the fulfilment of earthly destinies, when we have no home but merely a temporary asylum on earth, this obviously is only a particular variant of the general feeling that life as a whole is an adventure. ... It stands outside that proper meaning and steady course of existence to which it is yet tied by a fate and secret symbolism. A fragmentary incident, it is yet, like a work of art, enclosed by a beginning and an end...like gaming, it contrasts with seriousness, yet, like the *va banque* of the gambler, it involves the alternative between the highest gain and destruction. (1959b: 248)

Whether, in the context of illness in the modern world, Broyard might have found Simmel's treatment of the adventure a mite too romantic is certainly arguable. But the idea that serious illness throws together activity and passivity (as fate), as well as conquest and grace, resonates with Gillian Rose's description of her cancerous existence as a 'life affair', making explicit the connection forged by Simmel between the love affair and the adventure. Both accentuate life, and in so doing, he said, are 'alien to old age', so that to find one's style in the face of illness suggests life-affirmation. Most important for the discussion here is that Simmel saw the adventure not as a separate sphere to be enjoyed by the select, but as a potential that lies in all social practices, i.e. in every fragment. In the ordinary sphere of existence this potential is allowed to 'emerge and submerge' with everyday events, yet when

– as with serious illness – life is crossed 'by tensions so violent' that this potential gains mastery over the material through which it realises itself, life appears as adventure, and then might actively be fashioned as such.

This line of argument proposes works of illness to be exemplars of a way of being in the world. This should not be mistaken for a plea to see either paintings or accounts of illness as 'metaphors for life'. This option is only there by virtue of a *post hoc* reflection upon 'work' and 'life' as if they were two aspects of a figure of speech. While the illness experience is, in a sense, 'torn from life', its form is not co-terminus with the account or the picture, both of which extend beyond events in the mundane world of disease and continue beyond the end of treatment. In the case of narrative, the 'account as a whole' (the account as read) fashions a distinct world lived as a totality, and this is achieved by virtue of the transmutations of the ordinary that have been discussed above. What is 'adventure-like' in the account of illness is that unfolding of events and actions that, dealing with chance and necessity, exemplifies significant meaning about life and how one lives it.

One of the key issues, then, is the relationship between the illness account and the events that it describes. Seen as an aesthetic project, the account is just one communication (albeit a special one) in an ongoing reflection upon the illness condition. It exemplifies a world of illness – an imaginary sphere – that finds re-instantiation time and time again in various contexts and moments of the person's life. So, in describing a significant moment (one that captures something important about being ill), the ascetic discipline of narrative shows forth this essence in literary form. It is not that some aesthetic essence is carried over, or better described, but that the meaning is achieved by virtue of being symbolised in the way set out above. This is indeed a kind of construction, but the idea is not reducible to the narrative forms or rhetorical devices that are essential for the achievement of ascetic distance, on which an aesthetic projection depends. Such a view separates the material and sensuous from the linguistic, so that the constructionist answer is given prior to, rather than following the analysis.

Frame Work: beside medicine and society

Earlier on in this chapter I raised the question, how do stories and paintings direct viewers and readers to the fact that they are doing a particular kind of representational work? In order to address this issue I shall draw upon an essay by Jonathan Bordo (1996) in which he makes the distinction between two uses of the word 'frame', as applied to contemporary art. In order to retain the clarity of Bordo's analysis, I will, for the moment, restrict my reference to artworks, extending it later on to photographs and text relating to illness. Following Benjamin (1970), Bordo argues that, for an art object to retain its aura (its mystery), it must remain within a context or niche that restricts its movement and its visibility. This is, in Benjamin's terms, the 'shell' from which an object can be 'pried' by the processes of universalization (and hence, commodification). This frames the artefact in the sense of culturally binding it, this being an act of symbolic closure.

Bordo argues that this sense of the word 'frame' (*parergon*) is inadequate to embrace certain kinds of artworks that make their claim to signify by eschewing what might be thought of as institutional contexts, and indicating their 'niche' within the work itself. This involves a kind of 'inner framing'. He uses the example of a sculptural display – the *Aboriginal Memorial* – to be found in the National Gallery of Australia. This comprises some two hundred inscribed poles that bear the name 'Hollow-Log Bone Coffins'. Each one represents or stands for a hollowed out tree trunk in which would be held the bones of Aboriginal people. While the context of the gallery is obviously relevant to the sculpture being seen as art (the first sense of frame), Bordo is interested in the work that must be done to make what appear to be actual objects into a signifying whole. His proposal is that this is made possible only by the thing – the hollow log – first being removed from its original niche, the cemetery of the aborigines. 'Only then can it operate as a signifying object that can stand metaphorically for a bone coffin and not *be* a bone coffin' (1996: 188, emphasis in original). Or in Goodman's (1968) terms, only then can it exemplify properties that it *metaphorically*, but does not *actually* possess. To remove is to make a replica, and it is the copy that signifies the mysteries of Aboriginal death. For the object to signify, it already has to *be* a replica, thus making it an icon. This act of self-reference involving a signifying copy constitutes an act of inner framing that is different to the frame that sets something off from its context, the idea of *parergon*. Inner framing involves self-reference that is fundamental not only to the way that works of illness signify, but also to their relationship to medicine and to the everyday world of ill people.

This second kind of framing involves, as well as replication, a de-positioning away from the niche in which the original possesses, using Benjamin's vocabulary, its auratic status, its mystery. The mystery in our case is, of course, pain and suffering. The niche might be a place or condition in which the person or object is conventionally found or understood, be it in the clinic or in the home; or it might be a schedule of comportment – a conventional way of acting. In the case of works of illness, de-positioning as replication often involves the person's bodily appearance being either removed from context or, as with the examples discussed previously, re-enacted. All performative art involving the body fits this condition, especially the work of people like Hannah Wilke and Jo Spence, who photographed themselves transgressively (outside the conventional niche) using devices of pose and theatre (Jones, 1998). Indeed much of what has been termed 'meta-communication' – which is nothing if not framing – depends upon presenting a message of the kind, 'this nip which denotes a bite does not denote what a bite would normally denote' (Bateson, 1987: 180). Discussing the communication of play by monkeys, Bateson described the nip as a sign of change in the mode of relating – to be read as 'this is play'. The essential point is not just that the nip *denotes* a bite differently, but that it is *part of the display* that exemplifies a mode of being (playfulness) that can be referred back as a descriptor of the performance. In establishing 'this is play', the nip comes to contextualise (the first meaning of frame, as 'contextually setting off') the sphere of play, but does this only through first indicating, presentationally and self-referentially, 'THIS is play' (the second meaning of framing). (This analysis extends to all similar forms of interaction, for example, flirting [Radley, 2003]).

We might, then, consider the following performance as involving framing, if not of art, then certainly of illness. It is described in a piece in the *San Francisco Chronicle* in 1999, as told by Jon Carroll, who had been helping at a parade:

> One image stands out: In the middle of all the revelry, the floats with the dancing boys and the dykes on bikes and the massed contingents of proud parents of gay children, a single woman marched down the middle of Market Street. She was bare to the waist. She had a mastectomy scar. She did not (in my memory at least) carry any sign or provide any instructions on how to view her presence – she was testifying on her own terms. ...
>
> I do not know her name. I have thought of her often. The more I remembered her, the more I decided that she had to be, for me, the image of the century....
>
> She confronted all her demons. She said: This is what a mastectomy looks like. Not as bad as your fears, not as bad as your ignorance, not the end of the world....
>
> I cannot pretend to understand the psychological impact of all this. Words do not convey that much. I can understand the issue in a dry political or social sense; that's as far as my brain takes me....
>
> And that is why that single image keeps coming back. It transcends reason and speaks to the heart. That marching woman, head up, eyes bright, her lips an enigmatic line – she speaks candidly about the reality

of pain and loss, and she says also: I am a woman. I am still real. I am your mother or your daughter. Deal with me. Love me. I am among you now; I always have been. (Carroll, 1999).

I cite this because of its simplicity of observation rather than its commentary. It illustrates the act of framing as de-positioning through performance, involving figurative display (walking bare to the waist) that signified illness by including a trace (the scar) of the territory (the demons) that she had traversed. The woman carried no sign for the simple reason that she configured it with her body. The trace was the mastectomy scar, an instance of what Bordo mentions as being paradoxical for contemporary art, 'things that have been deliberately fabricated as traces and yet seem to endanger the very trace quality of the sign that is the focus of fabrication' (1996: 184). (More familiar examples of this would include 'found objects' placed in galleries, whose claim to be art is always hotly contested.)

An example of such a trace can be found in the work of the artist Hannah Wilke, who photographed (amongst other pictures) locks of her hair that had fallen out due to the effects of chemotherapy on her body. (See Figure 17). Wilke's previous work had valorised qualities that she physically possessed, namely her physical beauty, a 'dangerous trace' indeed. It was her physical beauty that led to repeated criticisms of her earlier work – that she exploited her attractiveness, falling back into her niche as a glamorous woman – which criticisms were undone with the *Intra-Venus* series of photographs in which she continued to perform after being diagnosed with cancer. In this later work she photographed herself (or had herself photographed) nude, in glamour poses, without hair, her body bloated from the effects of her cancer.

Analysing her work, the art historian Amelia Jones has pointed out that Wilke's lasting aim was to pervert the logic of the male gaze by it being, 'unmoored from its conventional assumption of a priori fact and *reiterated* as conditional, motivated, and explicitly patriarchal' (1998: 153, emphasis in the original). This work of 'unmooring', of freeing from a niche, is made possible by a re-routing of signs, in which the depositioning of trace objects plays a central role.

Traces, therefore, are not just physical aspects or properties of places but involve conventional understandings that include expected ways of viewing. As mentioned above, it was feminists, rather than the public in general, who criticised Wilke for making pictures that could be viewed as glamour pictures, and thereby betraying the cause of progressive politics. This is an illustration of how de-positioning that deliberately problematizes the trace – endangering

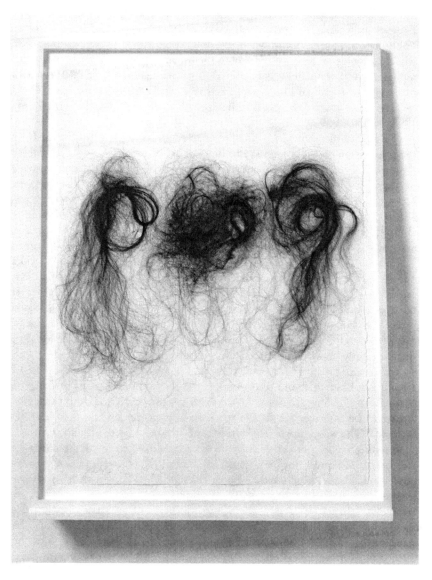

Figure 17. *Hannah Wilke "Brushstrokes No. 6: January 19, 1992",*
1992 artist's hair on arches paper 33 x 25 1/2 inches (F) Photo: Dennis Cowley,
Courtesy Donald and Helen Godard and Ronald Feldman Fine Arts, New York

its work of framing – puts in question whether the picture is to be taken ironically or literally. Only when Wilke photographed herself with cancer, using the same techniques that she had always employed, did she undo the remnants of glamour that had adhered to traces made in her earlier work. In that way, her works of illness came, retrospectively and posthumously, to act as a cultural frame (*parergon*) for her previous photographs as well (Barry, 1998; Knafo, 2000).

We saw earlier how Jo Spence re-enacted (in Jones's terms, *reiterated*) in her photographs what it was like to be treated in hospital for cancer, making these copies stand for the experiences that she underwent. The trace in many of these photographs is, paradoxically, the breast that was never to be removed, indicated sometimes with a cross to mark its status as signifier (see Figure 3, *Property of Jo Spence?*, p.69). In the picture *I Framed my Breast for Posterity*, (see Figure 2) the wooden frame that surrounds her breast is ironically a cultural closing device ('a picture of my breast') that also serves to 'frame' self-referentially. That is, it serves to de-position the whole scene in a quite radical way. Her partial nudity interrupts the domestic niche – effectively removes Spence from a conventional viewing – to establish her pose as performative, figurative and signifying. The trace (the threatened breast – a 'would be' trace) is shown as a sign feature referring to the fear of mastectomy and the horror of both its necessity and its consequences. The trace is clearly important in its status as symptom and sign, as being in effect, an accident re-made. The power of this photograph is amplified by the use of a culturally binding frame (the wooden picture frame Spence is holding) as part of a self-referential framing act. This makes ambiguous the trace (the 'breast to be removed') with the result that its power to lure the viewer is increased. The word 'frame' in the title carries both of these meanings.

Framing in the performative sense does not have to involve pictures of the body, although the body, in its mysteries of suffering, is always implicated. Martha Hall's artist's book *The Rest of My Life* is made up of de-positioned appointment cards, so that while these are the actual cards sent by the clinic, her act of binding them into the form of an artist's book 'pries them from their clinical niche', to paraphrase Benjamin. While physically the same cards, they are no longer 'the same'; they are, in Bordo's sense of the term, replicas (they 'pose' as appointment cards). This work of re-figuring *that the assembled cards do* is the precondition for the book to locate the sign of the frame on traces that are deposited (including the writing on the cards, the dates, as well as the actual tablets of medication). These implicate the world of medicine to which the book refers. And like Spence's photograph *I Framed my Breast for Posterity,* Hall's *The Rest of My Life* frames in both of the ways discussed. The cards are literally bound using medical bandaging, and set off as a distinct object by being placed in a clamshell box with ribbon ties. (Several of Hall's other books are boxed in this way.) Finally, being labelled as 'an artist's book' completes a series of cultural bindings that contextualise it – thus framing as *parergons* or contexts. One might add that depositing Hall's work in the libraries of universities further adds to their cultural binding as artist's books, subjecting them to restrictions in viewing and access that are part of the aura of this niche in which they are placed. This is an example of how cultural framing might affect, perhaps even neutralise, though cannot remove the potential of self-referential framing that is the book's exemplary work. On this point, it has been argued that exhibiting artworks in a gallery is to force them to undergo 'a kind of aesthetic convalescence' (Smithson, quoted in Bordo, 1996: 189).

Do stories of illness – as well as paintings and photographs – frame in this performative way? Not all perhaps, but those that are works of illness in the sense used here most certainly do. To repeat what has been said before, this is to be found in those 'touching non-narrative passages' (Riessman, 1990) that often report, through direct speech, what was said and seen at a particular time. In the case of texts, de-positioning can be indicated denotatively, by pointing directly to changes in mood. As well as this, self-reference is made explicitly, using deictic devices to indicate style in ways that foreground the author's mode of action. In the act of depositing traces to which the message refers, texts do this by including direct speech and metonymic devices that we have seen 'bring the present to the past'. Scars – both literal and metaphorical – that can be shown or depicted in pictures have to be *placed* in texts, often through forms of description (including direct speech) that move the reader by implicating them in an act of witness. To speak of a passage in a text as 'touching' is to recognise that what is shown is shown *to someone*, and that its purpose is only achieved with the recognition of what has been shown.

We might say that the act of framing is only comprehensible once one conceives of the viewer/reader as endorsing or accepting the artist or author's invitation to 'take aside' the realities of depiction. In a sense, the work only properly appears once the viewer/reader recognizes the invitation in the artist's gesture. Whether or not we wish to call this a 'taking over' of expressive gesture is less important than the recognition that to understand a work of illness is, first, to endorse it and only then to name it.

This returns us to the fact that works of illness are testimonies, and the act of framing is only partially understood without recognising this conclusion. Bordo puts forward a view that brings the analysis of framing even closer to how works of illness create shared meaning. This is based upon Wittgenstein's (1963) example of the imaginary culture in which every person has a 'beetle' in a box but everybody has access to (can see) only their own 'beetle'. (What is especially relevant here is that Wittgenstein was using this example to address the issue of the privacy of pain sensation.) He concluded that, even with the prohibition of inspecting each other's 'beetle', this would not result in the elimination of the word 'beetle', though it no longer is the name of a thing. The object as referent drops away with the box as container being the only visible representation of what is or only might be inside. Wittgenstein emphasises that his language game is not meant to show that pain does not exist, but that the use of denotation should not be taken as proof that there is a thing here to denote.

Similarly, there is 'no thing' where suffering is concerned, but this does not mean that there is 'nothing': a different way of signifying is called for.

Referring back to his example of the Hollow-Log Bone Coffins, Bordo argues that these containers are referents in a system where their original objects (bones) are similarly unavailable for inspection. What the artwork *Aboriginal Memorial* represents is clearly not the object that actual bone coffins (in their niche) would represent (i.e. 'this container that denotes a bone coffin does not denote what a bone coffin would normally denote'), for the reason that the container, as artwork, *does not refer to an object at all*. Play, death, and suffering are not objects to which one can point, or which can be made visible.

> This structure of representation is defined through the testamental character of the work where the object… is the visible stand-in for that which is outside and unrepresentable, for which the proxy is the visible sign. In this respect, testamental representation not only resembles the discourse of the sublime – for that which is pictured is itself a sign with respect to the unpicturable – but the discourse of the sublime is a special articulation of such testamental representation. (Bordo, 1996: 199).

With reference to Martha Hall's book *Jane, with Wings*, (see Figure 10, p. 120) the unfolding of the pages from outer to inner fold, leading ultimately to the injunction to the reader to close the book without knowing, can be regarded as an 'invitation to failure' on the part of the reader. This failure involves the impossibility of seeing Hall's experience of illness, of it being spelled out so as to objectify and bind it. For readers to be made to fail in this way, perhaps time and time again, is perhaps for them to realise the futility of this exercise and is the beginning of a sense that something else is being asked of them instead.

The work of internal framing, (to distinguish it once more from frame as cultural context) is to indicate how traces are to be made referents in pictures or books in order that the whole might be read with respect to what cannot be explained. In the case of the example of the *Aboriginal Memorial*, Bordo concludes that this work, consisting of 'a forest' of two hundred containers, refers to and is in turn understood in terms of what cannot be depicted – the aboriginal dead. If we refer this example to works of illness, we see that the proxies of posing bodies and transposed objects, together with the depiction of traces from the sphere (niche) of disease, together make possible a sign of an experience undergone, an 'accident' that happened. In the case of serious disease, this experience is communicable only as a passage through (a testimony to) what is unnameable. As a result, the meaning of such a work is traduced where we try to see it only as denoting some-thing. If this continues to happen then the work of internal framing is unrecognised, the reified trace becoming the locus for uncertainty, transgression and danger on the part of the viewer. The samples of Hannah Wilke's hair, fallen out as a result of her chemotherapy, can then become literal traces of treatment, the distasteful and unacceptable details of matters that should be abjected, kept private, removed. (Contrast this to the aura surrounding the relics of saints in previous centuries, or even of 'great men' such as Galileo, whose finger bone is still displayed in the National Museum of the History of the Sciences in Florence.)

Where the work of framing is recognised – is witnessed – then 'the visible keeps the invisible invisible, the name names the unnameable, just as the artwork as a replica preserves a void place for the undisclosable' (Bordo: 1996: 198). The void place is the condition of the illness experience, what in another context (to do with the Holocaust) has been described as 'the darkness that the language had to go through' (Felman, 1995: 34). In relation to works of illness, the idea of 'the darkness' does not resist meaning, nor is it a romantic description of what is just beyond reach, (except where one tries to *see* it). The eradication of the void – of the patient's experience – is not without its advantages, of course. Modern medicine is built upon making the body accessible through the use of observation, palpation and the invention of the stethoscope. Recent developments in endoscopy, in genetic analysis and tissue management bring pathology closer, defines it more clearly. What underlies these developments continues to be the exclusion of darkness, as in the origin of modern medicine:

> ... ear and hand are merely temporary, substitute organs until such time as
> death brings to truth the luminous presence of the visible; it is a question of

mapping in life, that is in *night*, in order to indicate how things would be in the white brightness of death. (Foucault, 1973: 165, emphasis in the original).

This kind of luminescence – *the white brightness of death* – is gained at the expense of marginalizing the darkness that living with illness involves. It is not surprising, therefore, that at the present time, with changes to the authority of medicine, stories, paintings and photographs about illness should find themselves subject to both interest and subjugation.

What this brief analysis shows is that some of the works of illness discussed so far achieve their effect through a kind of internal framing that is central to both their testimony and to their being witnessed. This kind of framing works alongside *parergon*, the cultural contexts that tell us that a picture is a picture, that what is inside is separated from outside and to be treated differently. These cultural frames as boundaries are strong in the case of Robert Pope's pictures and Jackie Stacey's book *Teratologies*. Pope's pictures were made in hospital, and while they are expressive of illness and care, they make depictions of hospital scenes (the niche or setting) using, with awareness, aesthetic devices from the world of art. Jackie Stacey's book is set in the context of academic publishing, so that the stories she tells about her illness are contained within the dominant frame of intellectual analysis that conceptualises her own and other people's cancers. Autobiographical stories, such as those by Frank, Rose and Broyard, are not without analytic reflection (if anything, this adds to their power). However, each of these authors provides both a proxy (the figure in the story) and includes traces deposited as an internal niche. For example, Rose provides a rare description of what it is like to live with a colostomy; Frank gives details of his treatment, and Broyard relates details of how cancer colours his everyday life.

Given these differences between works, it is not my intention to say – as in an empirical exercise – that all stories and pictures about serious illness use internal framing in the ways discussed above. And yet, insofar as these works need to instantiate a place (a niche) from which to testify about what is unnameable, and to indicate to the witness how the work should be read – in short, to make its meaning by declaring itself to be an exemplar of that incidence – then these works need to be understood to be engaged in internal framing. Unless we distinguish this work from cultural binding (framing as closure) then any further discussion of the relationship of works of illness to medicine, art and the everyday world is likely to be incomplete, if not in error.

Without the Frame

To build on the idea of internal framing, or to go back to its links with changes in art in the last fifty years, is to see that works of illness are already critical in being ready to position themselves beside the authority of medicine, art or science. The idea of framing was discussed earlier in terms of testimony and witness, as well as aesthetics and the sublime. While it is possible to speak of works of illness in terms of what they do, or how they signify, it is less easy to do so from a perspective that takes them as if they formed a body of artefacts 'as a whole'. And this is what one is invited or tempted to do when moving to a discussion of the relationship of such works to medicine, art or social science. I hope enough has been said to see why these works are inadequately understood as flawed enterprises that fail to make the grade clinically, aesthetically and scientifically. Foremost surely, is the fact that they are created under different conditions, for different purposes, in different genres and are read and viewed in different contexts.

If we do seek for an overarching view, then works of illness might be thought of, figuratively, as symptomatic of changes taking place in each of these spheres. I have already mentioned certain technological developments in medicine that enhance its powers to discern the body and to monitor individuals at a distance. Using the comparison mentioned above, we might say that medicine has concentrated its beam of light so as to illuminate focally and yet to cast its beam more widely. The result of this is not merely to see some things better, but to throw other things into sharp relief while yet casting shadows that give shape to darkness. Without pressing this figure too far, what this means is that the issues that works of illness address are matters that medicine has created as an adjunct to its technological advance.

But this is not enough, for the reason that alongside this there has developed among some people a suspicion of scientific knowledge and of technological advances. This has occurred even as the latest consumer gadgets are snapped up in the course of enhancing or self-monitoring one's health, whether this is gym equipment for the home or blood pressure machines for daily use. What we think of as the environmental movement has a suspicion not only of what technology does to the 'natural' world, but also of the certainties that scientists use to justify risks involved. The appeal of alternative medicine lies in no small part in this attitude. When taken together with new medical treatments, the ways these are seen – for example, the 'slash and burn' description of treatments for breast cancer – provides the basis for resistance. In a world where the erosion of individual rights puts dignity at risk, patients may well refuse to contain their suffering within the niche allotted to them by modern medicine. The grounds for wanting to protest one's rights and the humanitarian shortcomings of a technologically driven medicine are set not necessarily by its most advanced applications, but by the indignities that are sometimes consequent upon them.

A photograph by Israeli artist Gideon Gechtman shows him standing, naked, with arms raised, displaying the scar from his heart surgery, and with all hair shaved from his head and body. Reporting a conversation with Gechtman about the picture, Barilan (2004) says that the removal of all body hair alludes to the occasion when Gechtman felt humiliated by having his pubic area shaved prior to surgery. While this is a common and easily understood pre-surgical requirement, the way that, as Barilan says, 'dehumanization is likely to crawl in the very moment' of care echoes once more that horror is not necessarily located in the primary incursion into the body (disease), but what comes on the back of its mundane consequences.

This gloss does not reduce Gechtman's photograph to a protest about being shaved, but points up the work of the trace in positioning the signifier outside of medical authority. Re-inserted into the cracks of institutional practices like these, works of illness draw attention away from the agency of medicine to the patient as territory and as the bearer of rights. This point is worth making because it underlines the fact that this is not primarily a critique of medicine in its aim to relieve suffering, but is instead a critique of a relationship that has lost what Frank (2004) calls its 'generosity'. One can see that these deficiencies in humanitarian treatment are not easily made significant by being added up as a series of instances, because indignity (like suffering) is opaque. And, to return to the example just discussed, pre-surgical shaving is, from a medical point of view, there to reduce risks of infection. In response to works with a critical edge, one can always say with the medical perspective: 'they are doing the best they can'.

I should discuss works of illness once more (if only briefly) in their relationship to the sphere of art as a cultural and commercial field. I said at the outset that, while this book is about the aesthetic potential of stories and pictures concerning illness experience, whether they are deemed to be art (with a capital 'A') is of secondary concern here. This proviso holds while one is discussing pictures, especially, in close relation to their locus of production, but becomes strained when considering them in their biography as artefacts. It is important to consider whether a work might be enhanced in its role as a signifier of illness or whether this role might be diminished. When making their photographs and artist's books, it was important both to Jo Spence and to Martha Hall to consider their *practice* as art rather than as something else. What this something else might be is unclear (but see below), the point being that what they made was something that was the product of ascetic distance and resulted in a product that stood up on its own. In addition, both women recognised the credibility and legitimacy accorded to work that has the label 'art'.

One of the developments in modern everyday culture is the growth in confessional display as entertainment and in a specular orientation to images that incorporate transgression. I have said that works like those of Spence and Wilke are not immune from this current but that neither is embraced by it. Both artists have 'something to say', not merely offering eye candy to the visually inquiring. It becomes possible, however, to see works that locate themselves by virtue of the traces they show – and this can include text as well as pictures – as merely distasteful. From what position are they distasteful? I think not from that of a modern, self-reflexive art, but from an intellectualised understanding of art that aestheticises the world. This position is also one that tends to moralise about the mass consumption of images as kitsch, the confessional as narcissistic. This is not to deny that this cultural stream exists (though perhaps not so populist as some might think) but to argue with Roberts (1998) that to reject everything that it touches risks falling prey to an anti-representational politics that is easily allied with censorship. It is on this ground, I think, that individuals who have made these works have risked their dignity, and have done this in order to show – *with indignation* – what they or others had gone through in the course of illness and its treatment. Whether removal – either temporarily or permanently – to a gallery legitimates what can be shown in such works is another matter. But there are risks here too, as when the popularity of the artist for other reasons obscures the message of the works created. One example of this is the work of Mexican artist Frida Kahlo, whose paintings have come to have a worldwide fascination enhanced by the circumstances of her biography. Indeed, it has been said that the representational significance of her works has been undermined by her celebrity status, so that when shown her paintings run the risk of being described as advertisements to her production of herself (for a rejection of this criticism and a defence of Kahlo's paintings, see Zarzycka, 2006).

To move works of illness into the context of the art world is to grant them another kind of existence, but at a price – their increased distance from the people for whom they might have been made. This also removes them from consideration by those who understand illness as a social phenomenon, perhaps most readily the sociologist of health, illness and medicine. For those of us (and here I include myself) who work in this field of study, representations that are fictional, autobiographic or visual provide difficulties of verification. It is perhaps the lack of procedures by which we can tell whether works of illness tell us the truth – and hence about their significance – that makes them problematic as sources of data. But as I hope to have shown, to treat them in this way is to misunderstand if not the works themselves, then the role that they might play in furthering our understanding of health and illness. In part, this is the result of the separation of the everyday from spheres of knowledge to which I have aligned myself in making my argument here. If examined in detail, it can be shown that the procedures that people use for validating knowledge are not wholly exclusive by sphere, and that there are arguments for the validation of social science data in terms of trustworthiness (rather than truth), using exemplars as the basis of inquiry (Mishler, 1990).

It is possible to engage in a study of artworks, text or visual, by taking them as products made within society, their eventual form and value being the contribution of a number of institutions and individuals of whom the artist/author is but one agent (Becker, 1982). This kind of study might well provide useful information about works made in relation to illness, but it will fall short to the extent that it deliberately cedes all analysis of the aesthetic to the humanities (Zangwill, 2002). This falling short is arguably the price that sociology is willing to pay to remain grounded in a rational study of institutions, ideologies and practices, because the larger risk is to dabble in unnameable matters with which such works engage. And yet, having posited a postmodern condition for society, social scientists re-discover that cultural practices are being re-formed at the margins. People do this using whatever means they have available to represent their condition and to fashion ideas for alternative ways of living. In the case of illness this might mean organising fun-runs in support of breast cancer fund raising; it might also mean the many Internet sites, some of which use imagery on their web pages. And it might include the copying, transforming, sharing and distribution of texts and images relating to people's experience and what it means.

It has been said that, in the face of life's horror, there is only one comfort – 'its alignment with the horror experienced by previous witnesses' (Canetti, 1974). The mapping of another's experience on to one's own is, as we have seen, enhanced in its potential when that experience is figured aesthetically, as a work. There is much to be learned about the ways that the new illness sub-cultures operate, not least in the way that stories as well as pictures are used to make certain kinds of space, in which, to paraphrase Swidler (2001), 'everyone can see that everyone else has seen what they have undergone' – not to mention where they stand. In that case, testimony and witness come to the fore not to replace representation but, in their many and several readings and viewings, to enhance it. While it is not possible to generalise about works as a result of this it does mean that, to the extent that they continue to matter, they are immune from being quite absorbed into the fields of art, or medicine or science. They are not just for delight, or to be adapted as therapeutic instruments or even to provide rich and interesting data. Made in the interstices – as it were – between these spheres they are fugitive and yet resilient, to the extent, that is, that they retain their power to stand up, effectively *to be works.*

If stories and pictures about illness are indeed ways of staying alive for the individuals who make them, if they are icons for people with serious disease, and if they are talismans for people who wonder how they might face such events in the future, then they are arguably important in the changing relationship of medicine to society. The world where health meant 'not being ill' is fast declining for postmodern societies, if it has not vanished already. And with that change in the idea of health comes changes in the idea of illness. To be ill has been, for some while, contingent upon whether people have a chronic disease, so that how one bore one's illness pointed up moral and ethical issues that were not apparent for the patient with acute conditions, in their relationship to the doctor. The chronically ill patient was a person who had to adapt, live with, and negotiate the consequences of beneficial treatment that had saved life and could now maintain it. Illness became altogether a more complicated experience, through meeting the events in everyday life that, following treatment, turned the patient into a sufferer. Now, the reach of medicine as embodied in techniques of surveillance and monitoring promises the emergence of a further change, in which the individual is healthy to the extent that she is active in the anticipation of what she might do in the event of health failures. This is a step beyond the 'good practices' that being healthy demands in a consumer society. The question becomes, how should one create the conditions under which anticipated illness can be dealt with effectively and properly?

Works and the Everyday

Because works of illness problematise the dominant legitimacy of the spheres of medicine, science and art, they tend to re-figure the everyday world (Featherstone, 1992). The world of everyday life is the location for illness, concerning as it does bodily practice, care, an immersion in the immediacy of suffering, and the sociality of interpersonal engagements. The 'taken for grantedness' of this world makes it characteristically elusive to theory, though it yields to practice (to engagement within it) and in some respects (or in some quarters) to a *techne* that we might describe as style. The styles of the *flaneur*, the hero, or the adventurer are examples that come to mind here. These styles assume a shared cultural frame by which they might be recognised, so that actions carried out are seen as exemplary of a way of living.

The kinds of works considered in this book also depend upon the use of styles, though these are made possible by using recognised genres and devices that draw upon spheres of knowledge such as art and science. The aim of these works has been, in every case, to catch up the vernacular, the everyday in a way that makes it significant, that says to individuals who are similar, 'I am here too', and to others, 'recognise me for what I am'. And yet they cannot do this by erecting a theory or even a *techne* on the foundations of the everyday alone. It is the resistance to, the taking aside, and the essential borrowings from the dominant spheres that enable individuals to re-frame the everyday world. This re-framing transforms illness and suffering from the elusive (the ungraspable) to the elusory, the re-figured.

Reviewing the people whose work I have discussed in this book, not one of them appears only as a patient or sufferer. Every one of them stands with one foot in illness and the other in a sphere of knowledge and practice that they use to show the territory of which they would make us aware. Or rather, the works that they make stand in both realms, and must do so. Each one of these people re-discovers practice in the course of making the work; I argue this as opposed to saying that they merely apply their previous knowledge, though they do this too. I have talked about the way that Hannah Wilke and Jo Spence used their bodies to disturb assumptions about women and cancer. Arthur Frank, though writing as a sufferer about his cancer, does so in a way that is sensitive to the relationships of people to the institution of medicine, and goes on to use stories to reflect critically upon these. In a sense, out of Frank's attempt to tell his story is born his sociology. This is not a form of sociology merely in opposition to mainstream thought but one that borrows concepts (e.g. narrative, body) to establish a different way of thinking.

Gillian Rose's book, *Love's Work*, is a philosophical reflection about both her illness and her personal relationships, in which the telling of her story creates an internal frame in terms of which her everyday experiences make a particular sense. I do not want to labour this point except to say that in every case – Robert Pope, Jackie Stacey and Anatole Broyard included – the work draws upon some sphere other than the everyday to create its meaning. Of course, some have one foot more firmly in the expert sphere than others – Jackie Stacey's book for example, is an academic text in which her story is contained. Even Martha Hall's artist's books are discussed here because her work is collected in university libraries, and has become the subject for displays – still few, still modest, but undoubtedly framed as art.

The implication of this is that works made primarily *within the everyday* (not by unknown individuals) need to be brought to a specialist sphere if they are to be recognised. By this I do not mean merely known more widely, but seen to be works that exemplify freedoms that are only discernable 'under the laws' of art, or science or politics. On the one hand, the judgment about whether a particular picture or story 'is a work' – that it stands up on its own – requires criteria drawn from art, the humanities and possibly social science. On the other, the multiplication of mediators that are provided by re-contextualisation within a gallery, library or book is a condition not only for its recognition as a work, but in order that it can *do its work as* a narrative, *as* a painting, *as* a theatrical performance (Morris, 1998). So while it is important to recognise the emergence of works that problematise medical practice, scientific knowledge, or political hierarchies, it is equally important not to believe that they simply reflect the vernacular, or exemplify illness as an experience of the everyday. If works of illness are handles to grasp the 'unknowable', then they achieve this status only because they are drawn with a skilled hand moving in the darkness.

Of course there are works made by seriously ill people from within the everyday world, that draw upon art or literature in ways that specialists would regard as superficial or repetitive. Support groups, Internet discussion groups and the house magazines of specific cultures based on particular diseases abound with stories, poems and drawings, the fate of many remaining uncertain. My aim has not been to judge these products in that setting alone because, until they are brought within the sphere of art or letters, it is impossible to explore their potential as works. That is why I have not tried to examine a sample of stories or pictures made by patients selected at random. A sociological survey of this kind is entirely welcome but, if treated outside of the frame of medicine and art, is likely to miss how these works are positioned in relation to both of these spheres. The important point is that works of illness are *re-made* in social settings, in the course of social practices, in the varied and serial contexts in which they are exposed: they are not, in William James's words, products that come with labels on their backs.

To place a work in context is to extend its expressive potential through multiplying the mediation, which includes the opportunities for inspection or handling, the widening (or narrowing) of the audience, and its legitimation by inclusion within criteria of acceptability. But it is also to bring under the aegis of the work aspects of the context that it now inflects. The reproduction of paintings and the dissemination of stories through books and the Internet mean that the scope of works of illness is varied and extensive, involving contexts both private and public. For Arthur Frank (1991), it was a poster in his living room of a Biblical painting by Chagall, showing Jacob being blessed by the angel. This exemplified something that could inflect Frank's world, in a meaningful way, at a difficult time. Turn this round – the Chagall painting that had hung on his wall for some time 'waited' for the critical moment that marked Frank's trial of recovery from cancer.

Works of illness that 'stand up' do so not only because they are fashioned under the discipline of genres – even though they may turn these in the process. This is because they are resilient to viewings or readings across context, able to bring under their aegis the concerns or interests of those who consult them. This might be other people who suffer, it might be an audience of dispassionate readers or viewers, or it might be medical personnel. I am not saying here that such artefacts are interesting only to those who are already interested in what they have to say. Rather, they work by replicating, performatively, what Felman (1995) has called an 'accident' in the audience, which refers in this case to the accident of illness that befell the performer (artist or writer). Of course the audience do not fall ill, and there will be, as we have seen, a range of possible responses that are not predictable, because each viewing or reading is not another instance but a co-incidence of work and context. But those who are moved, enlightened or enraged by a story or painting about illness *fall* nonetheless, in the sense that they are lured into a territory – the figured space that works create – that in a sense then passes through them. The 'accident' might then re-appear in the form of witnessing, made possible by the figuration of the illness experience.

In conclusion, there seems little question that an increasing number of stories and pictures by seriously ill people have emerged over the last forty years or so. This period has seen the growth of social movements, some that resisted, others that tried to change the social order. And in the space of less than twenty years we have seen the rise and decline (some might say the transformation) of particular movements like ACT UP in its fight for the rights of people with AIDS. Alongside this there have been changes in the genres, in styles of expression, and in the cultural forms of mediated entertainment and information. Works of illness – as with all artworks – are contingent upon mediated practices of representation, production and consumption. As I have acknowledged, one cannot talk about works outside of these developments, or imagine that they defy the historical and social currents that gave rise to them and influenced their consumption. However, it would be short-sighted to think that we can understand serious illness without addressing how it is rendered sensible, which work includes aesthetic as well as political and moral endeavours.

References

Abbas, A. (1989) On fascination: Walter Benjamin's images, *New German Critique*, 48, 43-62.

Adamson, C. (1997) Existential and clinical uncertainty in the medical encounter: an idiographic account of an illness trajectory defined by Inflammatory Bowel Disease and Avascular Necrosis, *Sociology of Health and Illness,* 19, 133-59.

Adorno, T.W. (1984) *Aesthetic Theory.* Trans. C. Lenhardt. G Adorno and R. Tiedemann (eds.), London: Routledge and Kegan Paul.

Arendt, H. (1973) *On Revolution.* Harmondsworth: Penguin.

Atkinson, P. (1997) Narrative turn or blind alley? *Qualitative Health Research,* 7, 325-344.

Atkinson, P. and Silverman, D. (1997) Kundera's *Immortality*: the interview society and the invention of the self, *Qualitative Inquiry,* 3, 304-325.

Australian Broadcasting Corporation (2006) Sunday Morning - The Critics part 6: Arlene Croce - 27/11/2005. http://www.abc.net.au/rn/arts/exhibita/stories/s1516830.html] (Consulted 4 July 2006)

Barilan, M. (2004) Medicine through the artist's eye: before, during and after the Holocaust, *Perspectives in Biology and Medicine*, 47, 110-134.

Barry, J. (1998) Living with contradictions – Hannah Wilke, *Journal of the International Association of Physicians in AIDS Care*, 4, 28-34.

Barthes, R. (1977) *Image Music Text: Essays*. Selected and translated by Stephen Heath. London: Fontana Press.

_____ (1982) *Camera Lucida: reflections on photography*. Trans. Richard Howard. London: Jonathan Cape.

Bateson, G. (1987) *Steps to an ecology of mind*. Northvale, NJ: Jason Aronson.

Batt, S. (1994) *Patient No More: The Politics of Breast Cancer*. London: Scarlet Press.

Becker, H.S. (1982) *Art Worlds*. Berkeley: University of California Press.

_____ (1988) Visual sociology, documentary photography, and photojournalism: It's (almost) all a matter of context. In J. Prosser (ed.) *Image-based research: a sourcebook for qualitative researchers*. London: Falmer Press. pp 84-96.

Bell, S.E. (2002) Photo images: Jo Spence's narratives of living with illness, *health: An Interdisciplinary Journal for the Social Study of health, Illness and Medicine*, 6, 5-30.

_____ (2004) Beyond texts: Layers of meaning in the videodiary "A healthy baby girl", Presented to the American Sociological Association Annual Meetings, August 16, 2004, San Francisco, CA. p. 12.

_____ (2006) Living with breast cancer in text and image: making art to make sense, *Qualitative Research in Psychology* 3, 31-44.

Benhabib, S. (1990) Hannah Arendt and the redemptive power of narrative, *Social Research*, 57, 167-196.

Benjamin, W. (1970) *Illuminations*. Ed. H. Arendt, trans. H. Zohn. London: Jonathan Cape.

_____ (1933/1979) Doctrine of the similar, *New German Critique*, 17, 65-69.

_____ (1986) 'One -way street'. In P. Demetz (ed.) *Reflections: essays, aphorisms and biographical writings*. New York: Schocken Books. pp 61-94.

Berger, J. (1991) *About looking*. New York: Vintage Books.

Berger, J. and Mohr, J. (1989) *Another way of telling*. Cambridge: Granta.

Bochner, A. (2001) Narrative's virtues, *Qualitative Inquiry*, 7, 131-157.

Bohls, E.A. (1993) Disinterestedness and denial of the particular: Locke, Adam Smith, and the subject of aesthetics, In P. Mattick, Jnr (ed.) *Eighteenth-century aesthetics and the reconstruction of art.* Cambridge: Cambridge University Press. pp16-51.

Boltanski, L. (1999) *Distant suffering: morality, media and politics.* Translated by G. Burchell. Cambridge: Cambridge University Press.

Bordo, J. (1996) The witness in the errings of contemporary art. In P. Duro (ed.) *The rhetoric of the frame: essays on the boundaries of the artwork.* Cambridge: Cambridge University Press. pp 178-202.

Bowler, A.E. (1997) Asylum art: the social construction of an aesthetic category. In V.L.Zolberg and J.M.Cherbo (eds.) *Outsider Art: Contesting boundaries in contemporary culture.* Cambridge: Cambridge University press. pp 11-36.

Braun, L. (2003) Engaging the experts: popular science education and breast cancer activism, *Critical Public Health,* 13, 3, 191–206.

Breast Cancer Fund (1998) *Art.Rage.Us.: The Art and Outrage of Breast Cancer,* San Francisco: Chronicle Books.

Breast Cancer Fund (2000) "Obsessed with Breasts" Ad Campaign. http://www.breastcancerfund.org/site/pp.asp?c=kwKXLdPaE&b=83016 [Accessed 27 June 2006]

Brown, P., Zavestoski, S., McCormick, S., Mayer, B., Morello-Frosch, R. and Altman R.G. (2004) Embodied health movements: new approaches to social movements in health, *Sociology of Health and Illness,* 26, 50-80.

Broyard, A. (1992) *Intoxicated by my illness: and other writings on life and death.* New York: Fawcett Columbine.

Buck-Morss, S. (1992) Aesthetics and Anaesthetics: Walter Benjamin's Artwork Essay reconsidered, *October,* 62, 3-41.

Burke, E. (1759/1990) *A Philosophical Enquiry.* Oxford: Oxford University Press.

Bury, M. (1982) Chronic illness as biographical disruption, *Sociology of Health and Illness,* 4, 167- 82.

Butler, S. and Rosenblum, B. (1991) Videotape. *Cancer in Two Voices.* Lucy Massie Phoenix and Annie Hershey (Eds.) Sandbar Productions.

_____ (1994). *Cancer in Two Voices.* London: The Women's Press.

Caillois, R. (1984) Mimicry and legendary psychasthenia, *October,* 31, Winter, 17-32.

Canetti, E. (1974) *Kafka's other Trial.* New York: Schocken.

Carroll, J. (1999) 'The image of the century'. *San Francisco Chronicle*, Friday 31 December.

Carson, R.A. (1995) Beyond respect to recognition and due regard. In S.K.Toombs, D. Barnard and R.A. Carson (eds.) *Chronic Illness: from experience to policy*. Bloomington: Indiana University Press. pp 105-128.

Cartwright, L. (1998) Community and the public body in breast cancer media activism, *Cultural Studies*, 12, 117-138.

Caruth, C. (1996) *Unclaimed experience: trauma, narrative, and history*. Baltimore: Johns Hopkins University Press.

Cassell, E. (1972) Being and becoming dead, *Social Research*, 39, 528-542.

———— (1991) *The nature of suffering: and the goals of medicine*. New York: Oxford University Press.

Cavell, S. (1985) What photography calls thinking, *Raritan*, 4, 1-21.

Chandler, M. (1991) Voices from the front: AIDS in autobiography, *Autobiography Studies*, 6, 54-64.

Chaplin, E. (1994) *Sociology and visual representation*. London: Routledge.

Charon, R. (2006) *Narrative medicine: honoring the stories of illness*. Oxford: Oxford University Press.

———— (2009) Narrative medicine as witness for the self-telling body, *Journal of Applied Communication Research*, 37, 118–131.

Clarke, B. (1999) Why memoir isn't always art, *The Chronicle of Higher Education*, October 29, B9.

Coates, K.E. (2002) Exposing the "nerves of language": Virginia Woolf, Charles Mauron, and the affinity between aesthetics and illness, *Literature and Medicine*, 21, 242-263.

Cooper, P. (2002) 'Violence, pain, pleasure: *Wit*.' In T. Fahy and K. King (eds.) *Peering Behind the Curtain: disability, illness and the extraordinary body in contemporary theater*. New York: Routledge. pp 24-34.

Couser, G.T. (1991) Autopathography: women, illness and lifewriting, *Autobiography Studies*, 6, 65-75.

———— (1997) *Recovering Bodies: Illness, Disability and Life Writing*. Madison, Wisc.: University of Wisconsin Press.

Creekmur, C.K. (1996) Lost objects: photography, fiction, and mourning. In M Bryant (ed.) *Photo-textualities: reading photographs and literature*. Newark: University of Delaware Press, pp 73-82.

Crimp, D. (1992) Portraits of people with AIDS. In L. Grossberg, C. Nelson and P.A. Treichler (eds.) *Cultural Studies*. New York: Routledge.

Crimp, D. and Rolston, A. (1990) *AIDSDEMOGRAPHICS*. Seattle: Bay Press.

Croce, A. (1994/5) Discussing the undiscussable, *The New Yorker*, 26 December – 2 January, 54-60.

Cussins, A. (1992) Content, embodiment and objectivity: the theory of cognitive trails, *Mind*, 101, 651-688.

Deleuze, G. (1998) *Essays critical and clinical*. Trans. D.W.Smith and M. Greco. London: Verso.

Deleuze, G. and Guattari, F. (1994) *What is philosophy?* Trans. H. Tomlinson and G. Burchill. London: Verso.

Dennett, T. (2001) The wounded photographer: the genesis of Jo Spence's camera therapy, *Afterimage: the Journal of Media Arts and Cultural Criticism*, 29, (Nov/Dec), 26-27.

Diamond, J. (1998) *C: because cowards get cancer too...* London: Vermillion.

Diedrich, L. (2007) *Treatments: Language, politics and the culture of illness*. Minneapolis: University of Minnesota Press.

Dreuilhe, E. (1987) *Mortal embrace: living with AIDS*. Trans. Linda Coverdale, London: faber and faber.

Drucker, J. (1995) The century of artist's books, chapter 1, The artist's book as idea and form. New York: Granary Books. http://www.granarybooks.com/books/drucker2/drucker2.html (retrieved Nov. 15, 2004)

Dykstra, J. (1995) Putting herself in the picture: autobiographical images of illness and the body, *Afterimage*, 23, 16-20.

Elkins, J. (1996) *The Object Stares Back: on the nature of seeing*. San Diego: Harcourt Brace.

_____ (1999) *Pictures of the Body: pain and metamorphosis*. Stanford: Stanford University Press.

Engberg, K. (1991) Marketing the (ad)just)ed) cause, *New Art Examiner*, 18, 22-28.

Featherstone, M. (1992) The body in consumer culture, *Theory, Culture and Society*, 1, 18-33.

Felman, S. (1995) Education and crisis, or the vicissitudes of teaching. In C. Caruth (ed.) *Trauma: explorations in memory*. Baltimore: The Johns Hopkins University Press. pp 13-60.

Foster, H. (1985) *Recodings: art, spectacle, cultural politics*. Part Townsend, Washington: Bay Press.

Foucault, M. (1973) *The birth of the clinic: an archaeology of medical perception*. Trans. A.M. Sheridan Smith. London: Tavistock.

_____ (1980) In *Power/Knowledge: Selected interviews and other writings 1972-1977*. Colin Gordon (ed.) New York: Pantheon.

Frank, A.W. (1991) *At the will of the body: reflections on illness*. Boston: Houghton Mifflin.

_____ (1995) *The wounded storyteller: body, illness and ethics*. Chicago: University of Chicago Press.

_____ (1997) Illness as moral occasion. *health: An Interdisciplinary Journal for the Social Study of Health, Illness and Medicine*, 1, 131-48.

_____ (1998) Stories of illness as care of the self: a Foucauldian dialogue. *health: An Interdisciplinary Journal for the Social Study of Health, Illness and Medicine*, 2, 329-348.

_____ (2000a) The standpoint of storyteller, *Qualitative Health Research*, 10, 354-365.

_____ (2000b) Can we research suffering? Keynote Address, Sixth Annual Qualitative Health Research Conference, Banff, Alberta, April 6.

_____ (2004) *The renewal of generosity: illness, medicine and how to live*. Chicago: University of Chicago Press.

Frazer, J.G. (1959) *The Golden Bough: a study in magic and religion*. London: Macmillan.

Furedi, F. (2004) *Therapy culture: cultivating vulnerability in an uncertain age*. London: Routledge.

Galassi, P. (1988) Introduction. In N. Nixon, *Nicholas Nixon: Pictures of People*. New York: Museum of Modern Art; Boston: Little Brown.

Gamson, J. (1989) Silence, death and the invisible enemy: AIDS activism and social movement 'newness', *Social Problems*, 36, 351-367.

Geertz, C. (1972) Deep play: notes on the Balinese cockfight. *Daedalus*, 101, 1-37.

Gerhardt, U. (1989) *Ideas about illness: an intellectual and political history of medical sociology*. Basingstoke: Macmillan.

Gilman, S. (1995) *Health and Illness: Images of difference*. London: Reaktion Books.

Goffman, E. (1976) *Gender advertisements. Studies in the Anthropology of Visual Communication*, 3, Whole number 2.

Goldstein, R. (1991) The implicated and the immune. In D. Nelkin, D. Willis and S. Parris (eds) *A Disease of Society: cultural and institutional responses to AIDS*. Cambridge: Cambridge University Press.

Goodman, N. (1968) *Languages of art: an approach to a theory of symbols*. Indianapolis: Bobbs-Merrill.

———— (1978) *Ways of Worldmaking*. Indianapolis: Hackett.

Gray, R., Sinding, C., Ivonoffski, V., Fitch, M., Hampson, A. and Greenberg, M. (2000) The use of research-based theatre in a project related to metastatic breast cancer, *Health Expectations*, 3, 137-144.

Greenslade, R. (1997) Heading towards the exit. *Guardian, Media,* 6-7, 11th August.

Griffin, G. (2000) *Representations of HIV and AIDS: Visibility blue(s)*. Manchester: Manchester University Press.

Grover, J.Z. (1989) Visible lesions: images of people with AIDS, *Afterimage*, Summer, 10–16.

Habermas, J. (1996) *The Habermas Reader*, William Outhwaite (ed.), London: Polity Press.

Hall, M.A. (2003) *Holding In, Holding On*. Catalogue to accompany exhibition, Mortimer Rare Book Room, Smith College.

Harris, S. (2001) The return of the dead: memory and photography in W.G.Sebald's Die Ausgewanderten. *German Quarterly*, 74, 379-391.

Harrison, M. (2005) *In Camera Francis Bacon: photography, film and the practice of painting*. London: Thames and Hudson.

Herzlich C. (1995) Modern medicine and the quest for meaning: illness as a social signifier. In M. Augé M and C. Herzlich (eds.) *The meaning of illness: anthropology, history and sociology*. London: Harwood, pp 151-173.

Hevey, D. (1992) *The Creatures time forgot: Photography and disability imagery*. London: Routledge.

Holden, S. (2000) When and how AIDS activism finally found its voice and power: critics notebook. *The New York Times on the Web*. http://www.nytimes.com/2000/12/01/arts/01CHOI.html December 1, 2000 [consulted 10 May 2005]

Hunter, I. (1992) Aesthetics and cultural studies. In L. Grossberg, C. Nelson and P.A. Treichler (eds.) *Cultural Studies*. London: Routledge, pp 347-372.

Hyde, L. (1999) *The Gift: imagination and the erotic life of property*. London: Vintage.

Jones, A. (1998) *Body Art/Performing the Subject*. Minneapolis: University of Minnesota Press.

Juhasz, A. (1995) *AIDS TV: identity, community, and alternative video*. Durham: Duke University Press.

Katz, A. and Shotter, J. (1996) Hearing the patient's 'voice': toward a social poetics in diagnostic interviews, *Social Science & Medicine*, 43, 919-931.

Klawiter, M. (2000) Racing for the cure, walking women and toxic touring: mapping cultures of action within the Bay area terrain of breast cancer. In L.K.Potts (ed.) *Ideologies of Breast Cancer: feminist perspectives,* Houndmills: Macmillan, pp 63-97.

_____ (2004) Breast cancer in two regimes: the impact of social movements on illness experience, *Sociology of Health and Illness*, 26, 845-874.

Klein, P. (1998) Insanity and the Sublime: aesthetics and theories of mental illness in Goya's *Yard with Lunatics* and related works, *Journal of the Warburg and Courtauld Institutes*, 61, 198-252.

Kleinman, A. (1988) *The Illness Narratives: suffering, healing and the human condition.* New York: Basic Books.

Kleinman, A. and Kleinman, J. (1997) The appeal of experience: the dismay of images: cultural appropriations of suffering in our times. In A. Kleinman, V. Das and M. Lock (eds.) *Social suffering*. Berkeley: University of California Press, pp 1-23.

Knafo, D. (2000) Hannah Wilke: the naked truth, *Gender and Psychoanalysis*, 5 (1) 3-36.

Koestler, A. (1964) The logic of the moist eye. In *The Act of Creation*. Chapter 12. London: Hutchinson.

Kristeva, J. (1982) *Powers of Horror: An essay on subjection*. New York: Columbia University Press.

Lacan, J. (1979) *The Four Fundamental Concepts of Psycho-Analysis*. Trans. Alan Sheridan, Harmondsworth: Penguin.

Langellier, K.M. (2001). 'You're marked': Breast cancer, tattoo and the narrative performance of identity. In J. Brockmeier and D. Carbaugh (eds.), *Narrative and Identity: Studies in Autobiography, Self, and Culture*. Amsterdam & Philadelphia, PA: John Benjamins.

Langellier, K. M. and Peterson, E. E. (2004) *Storytelling in everyday life*. Philadelphia, PA: Temple University Press.

Latour, B. (1988) Opening one eye while closing the other … a note on some religious paintings. In G. Fyfe and J. Law (eds.) *Picturing Power: visual depiction and social relationships*. London: Routledge.

_____ (1998) How to be iconophilic in art, science and religion? In C. Jones and P. Galison (eds.) *Picturing Science Producing Art*. New York: Routledge. pp 418-440.

Lorde, A (1980/1985) *The Cancer Journals*. London: Sheba Feminist Publishers.

Lowell, R. (1977) *Day by Day*. London: Faber and Faber.

Lynch, D. and Richards, E. (1986) *Exploding into Life*. New York: Aperture Foundation/Many Voices Press.

Lynch, M. and Edgerton, S.Y. (1988) Aesthetics and digital image processing: representational craft in contemporary astronomy. In G. Fyfe and J, Law (eds.) *Picturing power: visual depiction and social relations*. London: Routledge. pp 185-220.

Lyotard, J-F. (1984) The sublime and the avant-garde, *Art Forum*, 22, 36-43.

Maffesoli, M. (1991) The ethic of aesthetics, *Theory, Culture and Society*, 8, 7-20.

Mantel, H. (2004) *Giving up the ghost: a memoir*. London: Harper.

Matuschka (1993) Matuschka explains the NYT photo in her article "Why I did it". (originally appeared in *Glamour* magazine, November 1993). http://www.songster.nct/projects/matuschka/why./html [consulted 25 February 2005].

Mauss, M. (1966) *The gift*. London: Routledge and Kegan Paul

Mayes, S. and Stein, L. (1993) *Positive Lives: responses to HIV: a photodocumentary*. London: Cassell.

Mercer, K. (1994). *Welcome to the Jungle: New Positions in Black Cultural Studies*. New York and London: Routledge.

Merleau-Ponty, M. (1968) *The visible and the invisible*. Evanston: Northwestern University Press.

Mishler, E.G. (1990) Validation in enquiry-guided research: the role of exemplars in narrative studies, *Harvard Educational Review*, 60, (4), 415-442.

Mitchell, W.J.T. (1994) *Picture theory*. Chicago: University of Chicago Press.

Moore, S.E. (2008) *Ribbon Culture: Charity, Compassion and Public Awareness*. Houndmills: Palgrave Macmillan.

Morris, D.B. (1998) *Illness and culture in the postmodern age*. Berkeley: University of California Press.

Morrison, T. (1987) The site of memory. In W Zinsser (ed.). *Inventing the truth. the art and craft of memoir*. Boston: Houghton Mifflin. pp 101-124.

———— (1993) *Beloved*. London: Chatto and Windus.

Murray, T.J. (1994) Illness and healing: the art of Robert Pope. *Humane Medicine: A Journal of the Art and Science of Medicine*, 10 (3).

Nichols, B. (1991) *Representing reality: issues and concepts in documentary*. Bloomington: Indiana University Press.

Nietzsche, F. (2001) *The Gay Science.* B. Williams (ed.), trans. J. Nauckhoff. Cambridge: Cambridge University Press.

Nixon, N. (1988) *Nicholas Nixon: Pictures of People.* New York: Museum of Modern Art; Boston: Little Brown.

O'Toole, R. (1996) Salvation, redemption and community: reflections on the aesthetic cosmos, *Sociology of Religion,* 57, 127-48.

Oates, J. C. (1988) "Adventures in Abandonment" Review of *Jean Stafford: A Biography,* by David Roberts. *New York Times* Book Review 28 August 1988.

———— (1999) Art and "Victim Art". In *Where I've Been and Where I'm Going: Essays, reviews and prose.* New York: Plume.

Ogdon, B. (2001) Through the image: Nicholas Nixon's "People with AIDS", *Discourse,* 23, 75 - 105.

Ogonowska-Coates, H. and Robertson, I. (1998) *I Feel Lucky: interviews and photographs celebrating cancer survivors.* Booklet to accompany photo exhibition 'I Feel Lucky', Palmerston North, New Zealand, February - March, 1998.

Onwura, N. (1991) *The Body Beautiful* [videorecording]. New York: Women Make Movies.

Osborne, T. (1997) Review article: The aesthetic problematic, *Economy and Society,* 26, 126-46.

———— (1998) *Aspects of Enlightenment: Social theory and the ethics of truth.* London: UCL Press.

Parry, J. (1986) *The gift,* the Indian gift and the 'Indian gift'. *Man,* 21, 453-473.

Patten, M. (1998) The thrill is gone: an act up post-mortem (confessions of a former AIDS activist), In D. Bright (ed.) *The Passionate Camera: photography and bodies of desire.* London: Routledge. pp 385-406.

Patton, C. (1995) Performativity and spatial distinction: the end of AIDS epidemiology. In A. Parker and E. K. Sedgwick (eds.) *Performativity and Performance.* New York: Routledge.

Pitts, V. (2004) Illness and Internet empowerment: writing and reading breast cancer in cyberspace, *health: An Interdisciplinary Journal for the Social Study of Health, Illness and Medicine,* 8, 33-59.

Pope, R. (1991) *Illness and Healing: images of cancer.* Lancelot Press, Hantsport, NS: Lancelot Press.

Potts, L.K. (2000) Publishing the personal: autobiographical narratives of breast cancer and the self. In L. K. Potts (ed.) *Ideologies of Breast Cancer: feminist perspectives,* Houndmills: Macmillan, pp 98-127.

Prosser, J. (2007) Visual mediation of critical illness: an autobiographical account of nearly dying and nearly living, *Visual Studies*, 22, 185-99

Radley. A. (1999) The aesthetics of illness: narrative, horror and the sublime, *Sociology of Health and Illness*, 21, 778-796.

_____ (2002) Portrayals of suffering: on looking away, looking at, and the comprehension of illness experience, *Body & Society*, 8, 1-23.

_____ (2003) 'Flirtation'. In J. Coupland and R. Gwyn (eds.) *Discourses of the Body* London: Palgrave. pp 70-86.

Radley, A. and Bell, S.E. (2007) Artworks, collective experience and claims for social justice: the case of women living with breast cancer. *Sociology of Health and Illness*, 29, 366-390.

Radley, A. and Kennedy, M. (1997) Picturing need: images of overseas aid and interpretations of cultural difference, *Culture & Psychology*, 3, 435-460.

Radley, A., Mayberry, J. and Pearce, M. (2008) Time, space and opportunity in the outpatient consultation: 'The doctor's story', *Social Science & Medicine*, 66, 1484 -1496.

Radley, A. and Taylor, D. (2003a) Images of recovery: a photo-elicitation study on the hospital ward, *Qualitative Health Research*, 13, 77-99.

_____ (2003b) Remembering one's stay in hospital: a study in photography, recovery and forgetting, *health: An Interdisciplinary Journal for the Social Study of Health, Illness and Medicine*, 7, 129-159.

Rampley, M. (2000) *Nietzsche, aesthetics and modernity*. Cambridge: Cambridge University Press.

Rey, H.A. (1973). *Curious George*, New York: Houghton Mifflin.

Ricoeur, P. (1991) *A Ricoeur Reader: Reflection and Imagination*. M.J.Valdes, (ed.) New York: Harvester Wheatsheaf.

Riessman, C.K. (1990) Strategic uses of narrative in the presentation of self and illness: a research note, *Social Science & Medicine*, 30, 1195-1200.

_____ (2002) 'Doing Justice: positioning the interpreter in narrative work'. In W. Patterson (ed.) *Strategic Narrative: New perspectives on the power of personal and cultural stories*. Lanham: Lexington Books, pp 193-214.

Roberts, J. (1998) *The Art of Interruption: Realism, Photography and the Everyday*. Manchester: Manchester University Press.

Rose, G. (1995) *Love's work*. London: Chatto & Windus.

Rosenblum, B. (1991) 'I have begun the process of dying'. In J. Spence and P. Holland (eds.) *Family Snaps: the meanings of domestic photography*. London: Virago. pp 239-244.

Scarry, E. (1985) *The Body in Pain: the making and unmaking of the world*. New York: Oxford University Press.

Schweizer, H. (1997) *Suffering and the remedy of art*. New York: State University of New York Press.

Sekula, A. (1978) Dismantling modernism, reinventing documentary (notes on the politics of representation), *Massachusetts Review*, 19, 859–883.

Sharf, B.F. (1997) Communicating breast cancer on-line: support and empowerment on the Internet, *Women and Health*, 26, 65–84.

Shaw, P. (2006) *The sublime*. Abingdon: Routledge.

Shotter, J. (1981) Telling and reporting: prospective and retrospective uses of self-ascriptions. In C. Antaki (ed.), *The psychology of ordinary explanations of behaviour*. London: Academic Press.

Silvers, A. (1978) Show and tell: the arts, cognition and basic modes of referring. In S.S.Madeja (ed.) *The Arts, Cognition, and Basic Skills*. St Louis: CEMREL.

Simmel, G. (1959a) The handle. In K. H. Wolff (ed.) *Georg Simmel, 1858-1918: a collection of essays*. Columbus: Ohio State University Press.

_____ (1959b) The adventure. In K. H. Wolff (ed.) *Georg Simmel, 1858-1918: a collection of essays*. Columbus: Ohio State University Press.

_____ (1968) Sociological aesthetics. In K.P.Etzkorn, Trans. *Georg Simmel: The Conflict in Modern Culture and other Essays*. New York: Teachers College Press.

Sontag, S. (1961) *Against interpretation: and other essays*. New York: Octagon.

_____ (1978) *Illness as metaphor*. New York: Farrar, Straus and Giroux.

_____ (1979) *On photography*. Harmondsworth, Penguin.

_____ (1991) *Aids and its metaphors*. Published together with *Illness as Metaphor*. London: Penguin.

_____ (2003) *Regarding the pain of others*. London: Hamish Hamilton.

Spence, J. (1986) The sign as a site of class struggle: reflections on the works by John Heartfield,. In P. Holland, J. Spence and S. Watney (eds.) *Photography/Politics: Two*. London: Comedia. pp 176-186.

_____ (1988) *Putting myself in the picture: a political, personal and photographic autobiography*. Seattle: Real Comet Press.

_____ (1992) Cancer and the marks of struggle; an interview with Jo Spence. In Hevey, D. *The Creatures Time Forgot: Photography and Disability Imagery.* London: Routledge. pp 120-133.

_____ (1995) *Cultural sniping: the art of transgression.* London: Routledge.

Spivey, N. (2001) *Enduring Creation: art, pain, and fortitude.* Berkeley: University of California Press.

Stacey, J. (1997) *Teratologies: a cultural study of cancer.* London: Routledge.

Strawson, P.F. (1959) *Individuals: an essay in descriptive metaphysics.* London: Methuen.

Summers, D. (1991a) Real metaphor: towards a re-definition of the 'conceptual' image. In N. Bryson, M. Holly and K. Moxey (eds.) *Visual Theory: painting and interpretation.* London: Polity Press. pp 231-259.

_____ (1991b) Conditions and conventions: on the disanalogy of art and language. In S. Kemal and I. Gaskell (eds.) *The Language of Art History.* Cambridge: Cambridge University Press.

Swidler, A. (1995) Culture in action: symbols and strategies, *American Sociological Review*, 51, 273-86.

_____ (2001) What anchors cultural practices. In T.R. Schatzki, K. Knorr Cetina and Evon Savigny (eds.) *The Practice Turn in Contemporary Theory.* London: Routledge. pp 74-92.

Taussig, M.T. (1993) *Mimesis and Alterity: a particular history of the senses.* New York: Routledge.

Tester, K. (1997) *Moral Culture.* Lomdon: Sage.

Tomlinson, J. (1994) *Francisco Goya* y Lucientes *1746-1828.* London: Phaidon.

Tompkins, J. (1985) *Sensational designs: the cultural work of American fiction 1790-1860.* New York: Oxford University Press.

Updike, J. (1990) *Self-consciousness: memoirs.* London: Penguin.

Van Schaick, E. (1998) Palimpsest of breast: Representation of breast cancer in the work of Deena Metzger and Jo Spence, Schuylkill, 2, 1. Retrieved 19 June 2000, from http://www.temple.edu/gradmag/fall98/schaick.htm

Waskul, D.D. and van der Riet, P. (2002) The abject embodiment of cancer patients: dignity, selfhood and the grotesque body, *Symbolic Interaction,* 25, 487-513.

Weigel, S. (1996) *Body- and Image- Space: Re-reading Walter Benjamin.* London: Routledge.

Williams, G.H. (2000) Knowledgable narratives. *Anthropology and Medicine,* 7, 135-140.

Wittgenstein, L. (1963) *Philosophical investigations.* Trans. G.E.M. Anscombe, Oxford: Blackwell.

_____ (1979) *Remarks on Frazer's Golden Bough.* R. Rhees (ed.). Retford: Brynmill.

Woolf, V. (1994) On Being Ill. In A. McNeillie (ed.) *The Essays of Virginia Woolf. Volume IV, 1925-1928.* London: The Hogarth Press. pp 317-329.

Young, K. (2000) Gestures and the phenomenology of emotion in narrative, *Semiotica*, 131, 79-112

Zangwill, N. (2002) Against the sociology of the aesthetic, *Cultural Values*, 6 (4), 443-452.

Zarzycka, M. (2006) 'Now I live on a painful planet': Frida Kahlo revisited, *Third Text,* 20 (1), 73 – 84.

Author Index

Subject Index

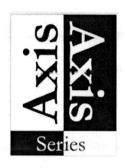

Series

Excessive Narratives
Georges Bataille, Self-Sacrifice &
The Communal Language of the Yucatec Maya
and U Chan Tsola'ni Ek Balam
Robert John Brocklehurst
September 2006 – 978-0-9551829-4-5
(April 2009 – 2nd Edition – 978-0-9556259-8-5)

Muse and Messiah
The Life, Imagination & Legacy of Bruno Schulz (1892 – 1942)
Brian R. Banks
December 2006 – 978-0-9551829-5-2
(April 2009 – 2nd Edition - 978-0-9556259-7-8)

Insect Nations
Visions of the Ant World from Kropotkin to Bergson
Simon King
December 2006 – 978-0-9551829-7-6

Fragmentary Futures
Blanchot, Beckett, Coetzee
Daniel Watt
June 2007 – 978-0-9551829-8-3
(April 2009 – 2nd Edition - 978-0-9556259 4 7)

Conceptual Breakthrough
Two Experiments in SF Criticism
James Holden and Simon King
December 2007 – 978-0-9556259-1-6

Souvenirs d'amour
Love and the mnemotechnic of alterity
(being fragments from an incomplete and interrupted dialogue)
Julian Wolfreys
December 2007 – 978-0-9556259-2-3

Student-Centred
Education, Freedom and the Idea of Audience
Neil Cocks
April 2009 – 978-0-9556259-6-1

Maciej Korbowa and Bellatrix
Stanisław Ignacy Witkiewicz
Translated and Introduced by Daniel Gerould
September 2009 – 978-0-9562749-1-5

Works of Illness
Narrative, Picturing and the Social Response to Serious Disease
Alan Radley
October 2009 – 978-0-9562749-0-8

CPSIA information can be obtained at www.ICGtesting.com
Printed in the USA
LVOW100948041111

253493LV00002B/98/P